Critical Care Focus

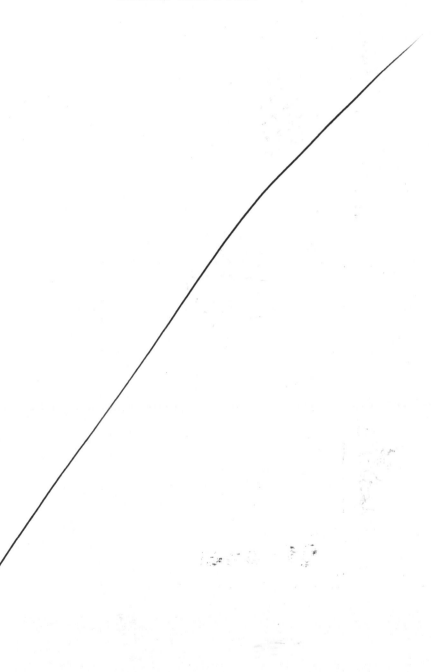

Critical Care Focus series

Also available:

H F Galley (ed) Critical Care Focus 1: *Renal Failure,* 1999.

H F Galley (ed) Critical Care Focus 2: *Respiratory Failure,* 1999.

H F Galley (ed) Critical Care Focus 3: *Neurological Injury,* 2000.

Critical Care Focus

4: Endocrine Disturbance

EDITOR

DR HELEN F GALLEY
Lecturer in Anaesthesia and Intensive Care
University of Aberdeen

EDITORIAL BOARD

PROFESSOR NIGEL R WEBSTER
Professor of Anaesthesia and Intensive Care
University of Aberdeen

DR PAUL G P LAWLER
Clinical Director of Intensive Care
South Cleveland Hospital

DR NEIL SONI
Consultant in Anaesthesia and Intensive Care
Chelsea and Westminster Hospital

DR MERVYN SINGER
Reader in Intensive Care
University College Hospital, London

BMJ Books   H0001388   WK100
             GALLEY

© BMJ Books 2000

BMJ Books is an imprint of the BMJ Publishing Group

First published in 2000
Second impression 2001
by BMJ Books, BMA House, Tavistock Square,
London WC1H 9JR

www.bmjbooks.com

British Library Cataloguing in Publication Data

A catalogue record for this book is available from the British Library

ISBN 0-7279-1582-7

Cover by Landmark Design, Surrey
Typeset by Phoenix Photosetting, Chatham, Kent
Printed and bound by Selwood Printing Ltd

Contents

Contributors

K George Alberti
Professor of Medicine and President of the Royal College of Physicians, London, UK

Irshad H Chaudry
Professor, Departments of Surgery, Molecular Pharmacology, Physiology and Biotechnology, and Director, Center for Surgical Research, Brown University and Rhode Island Hospital, Providence, Rhode Island, USA

Murad G Ghrew
Specialist Registrar in General Medicine and Intensive Care, Nuffield Department of Medicine, The John Radcliffe Hospital, Oxford

Charles Hinds
Consultant in Anaesthesia and Intensive Care, St Bartholomew's Hospital, London, UK

Paul Holloway
Consultant Chemical Pathologist in Intensive Care and Honorary Reader in Medicine, Nuffield Department of Medicine, The John Radcliffe Hospital, Oxford, UK

Martin G Schwacha
Assistant Professor, Department of Surgery and Center for Surgical Research, Brown University and Rhode Island Hospital, Providence, Rhode Island, USA

Greta Van den Berghe
Department of Intensive Care, Catholic University of Leuven, Belgium

Anthony P Weetman
Professor of Endocrinology, Department of Medicine, University of Sheffield, UK

Introduction

This is the fourth book in the series of 'State of the Art' volumes focusing on key issues in Critical Care Medicine. The series is taken largely from transcriptions of lectures given at Intensive Care Society meetings by renowned international experts. This issue of the series addresses endocrine problems encountered on the Intensive Care Unit and includes discussion of the endocrine disturbances seen during prolonged critical illness, the recent controversial growth hormone trials, a whistle-stop tour of diabetes for the intensivist and the influence of sex hormones on the immune and inflammatory responses.

Endocrine disturbances in prolonged critical illness

Greta Van den Berghe

Hypothalamic/anterior pituitary function, known to play a crucial role in normal metabolic and immunological homeostasis, is altered differently in acute and prolonged critical illness. This article provides an overview of the available data on this topic, focusing particularly on the somatotropic and thyroid axes.

Growth hormone therapy in the critically ill

Charles Hinds

Giving high doses of growth hormone to long-stay critically ill adults, at least during the first few weeks of their illness, is associated with increased morbidity and mortality. Although there are many publications in the literature since the mid-1950s in which growth hormone has been administered to catabolic patients without any suggestion of adverse effects, this unexpected finding emphasises the importance of continuing to perform prospective randomised controlled trials in critically ill patients, despite the difficulties inherent in designing, conducting and interpreting such studies. It is also clear that all randomised studies in intensive care patients should involve an unblinded safety committee.

Thyroid disturbance in the critically ill

Anthony P Weetman

Thyroid disturbance in the critically ill can lead to abnormalities in conventional thyroid function tests. These may confuse the unwary. Called sick euthyroid syndrome, this presupposes that these patients are truly euthyroid. However, this supposition has been challenged. The true, but rare, thyroid emergencies of thyrotoxicosis crisis and myxoedema coma are also discussed.

Diabetes for the intensivist

George K Alberti

This article provides an overview of diabetes, particularly in relation to those involved in care of the critically ill. Classification, diagnosis, risk factors, routine and emergency management of patients with diabetes are addressed.

Sex hormone-mediated modulation of the immune response after trauma, haemorrhage or sepsis

Martin G Schwacha, Irshad H Chaudry

Despite the fact that clinical studies have shown that gender affects morbidity and mortality after trauma, haemorrhage and sepsis, alterations in immune status under such conditions have been studied primarily in animals. Only recently have clinical studies begun to investigate the effect of gender, age, and sex hormones on immune response. In general, findings suggest that testosterone is immunosuppressive following traumatic injury, whereas the female sex hormones oestradiol and prolactin are protective under such conditions. The specific underlying mechanism(s) for the immunomodulatory properties of sex hormones on cell-mediated immune responses remains to be fully elucidated. Experimental evidence supports both direct and indirect effects in modulating the immune response.

The adrenal in critical care – do we neglect this vital organ?

Murad G Ghrew, Paul Holloway

In the absence of obvious clues to adrenal dysfunction, the management of patients on the intensive care unit may proceed without further specific attention to this organ, despite the vital role of the adrenal in the response to stress. The purpose of this article is to focus on the adrenal gland in critical care medicine, highlighting in particular the secondary effects of both critical illness and current intensive care therapies on adrenal function. In addition, the means at our disposal for diagnosing adrenal dysfunction and to appropriate management are discussed. The adrenal does not function as an independent endocrine organ and the relationship and dependency of the adrenal on the function of other organs, particularly the hypothalamus and pituitary are therefore also addressed. A recap of the range of homeostatic functions of the adrenal gland, and practical guidance on the evaluation and effective therapeutic compensation of adrenal function in critical care patients, are also provided.

1: Endocrine disturbances in prolonged critical illness

GRETA VAN DEN BERGHE

Introduction

Hypothalamic/anterior pituitary function, known to play a crucial role in normal metabolic and immunological homeostasis, is altered differently in acute and prolonged critical illness.[1] This article provides an overview of the available data on this topic, focusing particularly on the somatotropic and thyroid axes.

Hypothalamic growth hormone-releasing hormone (GHRH) is currently still considered to be the major endogenous and specific secretagogue for GH. Interaction between GHRH and the inhibitory hypothalamic factor somatostatin (SRIH) is thought to be responsible for the pulsatile pattern of GH secretion. In the past two decades, a series of synthetic GH-releasing peptides (GHRPs) and non-peptide analogues were developed and these have been found to potently release GH, through a specific G-protein coupled receptor located in the hypothalamus and the pituitary. Recently, an endogenous ligand of the GHRP-receptor has been discovered, labeled "ghrelin" which may be another key factor in the physiological regulation of pulsatile GH secretion.[2]

Acute changes within the growth hormone axis

(Figure 1.1)

During the first hours or days after an acute insult, circulating GH levels are elevated and the normal GH profile, consisting of peaks alternating with troughs at virtually undetectable concentrations, is altered: the amount of GH release from the somatotropes is increased, peak GH levels as well as interpulse concentrations are high and the frequency of GH pulses is increased. It is still unclear which factor ultimately controls the stimulation of GH release in response to stress. More frequent withdrawal of the

1

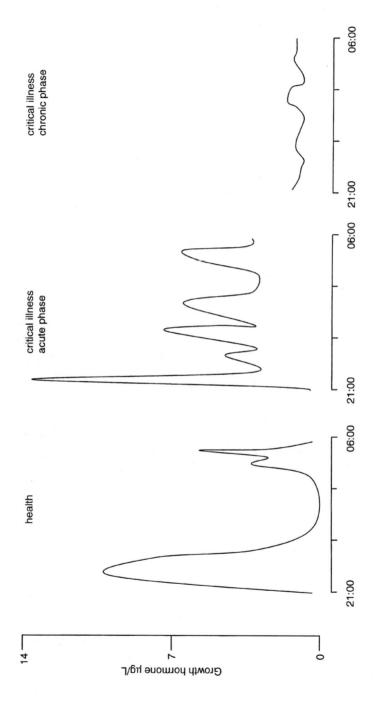

Figure 1.1   Nocturnal serum concentration profiles of growth hormone, illustrating the differences between the acute phase and the chronic phase of critical illness in the intensive care unit setting. Reproduced with permission from Van den Berghe G, de Zegher F, Bouillon R. J Clin Endocrinol Metab 1998;83:1827–34.[1]

inhibitory SRIH and/or an increased availability of stimulatory hypothalamic GH-releasing factors could hypothetically be involved. In addition, serum concentrations of insulin-like growth factor-1 (IGF-1) and the binding protein IFGBP-3 and its acid-labile subunit (ALS) decrease, preceded by a drop in serum levels of GH-binding protein (GHBP). The latter was found to coincide with reduced GH-receptor mRNA in peripheral tissues.[3] Circulating levels of the small (inhibitory) IFG-binding proteins are elevated. This situation has been interpreted as peripheral resistance to GH, although increased activity of IGFBP-3-protease in plasma also plays a role. It has been hypothesized – but it remains unproved – that the abundantly released GH during acute stress exerts direct lipolytic, insulin-antagonistic and immune stimulatory actions, while its indirect IFG-1-mediated somatotropic effects are attenuated.

Chronic changes within the growth hormone axis
(Figures 1.1 and 1.2)

If recovery does not follow within 7–10 days, intensive care support often may be needed for weeks or months. This chronic phase is characterised by a different set of changes in the somatropic axis.[4] Firstly, the pattern of GH secretion is chaotic and has a severely reduced pulsatile fraction and, although the non-pulsatile fraction is (still) somewhat elevated and the number of pulses is still relatively high, mean nocturnal GH serum concentrations are no longer substantially elevated, if at all. Secondly, pulsatile GH secretion correlates positively with circulating levels of IGF-1, IFGBP-3 and acid-labile subunit, which are all low. As low serum IGF-1 and – even more so – low levels of acid-labile subunit are markers of impaired anabolism in this condition, these findings suggest that a relative hyposomatotropism participates in the pathogenesis of the wasting syndrome seen characteristically in the chronic phase of protracted critical illness.[5] Male patients do worse than female patients in the sense that they lose more of the pulsatility and regularity within the GH-secretory pattern than women (despite indistinguishable total GH output) and also have lower IGF-1 and acid-labile subunit levels[6] (Figure 1.2).

Administration of growth hormone secretagogues
(Figure 1.3)

Studying GH responses to administration of GH secretagogues (GHRH and GHRP) enables – to a certain extent – differentiation between a primary pituitary and a hypothalamic origin of the relatively impaired GH release. The GH responses to GHRP in long-stay intensive care unit (ICU)

3

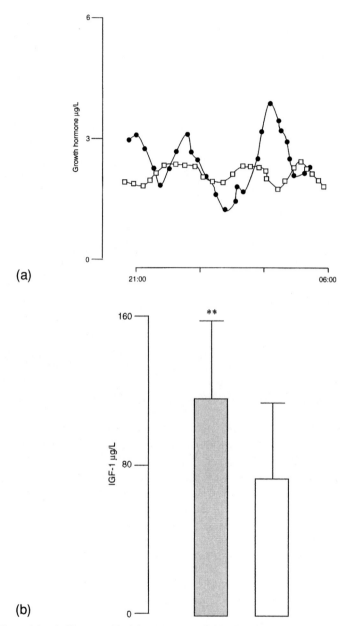

*Figure 1.2   A. The more "feminized" pattern of growth hormone secretion (more irregular and less pulsatile growth hormone secretory pattern for an identical mean nocturnal level) in prolonged critically ill men compared to women. Nocturnal growth hormone levels sampled every 20 minutes in a male patient (□) are shown compared to a matched female patient (●). B. Protractedly critically ill men also have lower insulin-like growth factor-1 concentrations than female patients. Mean + standard deviation. **p < 0.01. Adapted with permission from Van den Berghe G, Baxter RC, Weekers F, et al. J Clin Endocrinol Metab 2000;85:183–92.*[6]

4

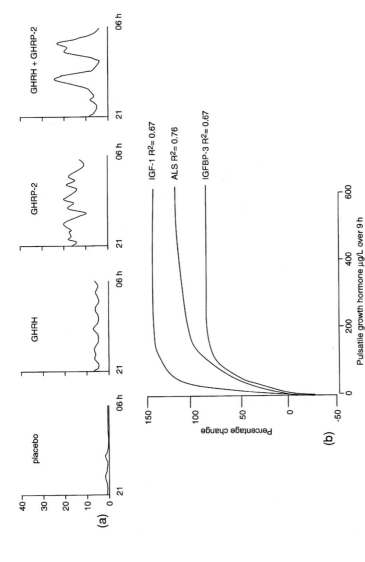

Figure 1.3   A. Nocturnal serum growth hormone (GH) profiles in the prolonged phase of illness, illustrating the effects of continuous infusion of placebo, growth hormone-releasing hormone (GHRH) 1 μg/kg/h; growth hormone-releasing peptide-2 (GHRP-2) 1 μg/kg/h; or GHRH + GHRP-2 1 μg/kg/h each. B. Exponential regression lines have been reported between pulsatile growth hormone secretion and changes in circulating insulin-like growth factor-1 (IGF-1), acid-labile subunit (ALS) and IGF-binding protein-3 (IGFBP-3) obtained with 45-hour infusion of either placebo, GHRP-2 or a combination of GHRH + GHRP-2. They indicate that the parameters of growth hormone responsiveness increase in proportion to growth hormone secretion up to a certain point, beyond which further increases in growth hormone have little additional effect. In the chronic phase of critical illness, growth hormone sensitivity is present, in contrast to the acute phase, suggesting growth hormone resistance. Reproduced with permission from Van den Berghe G, de Zegher F, Baxter RC et al. J Clin Endocrinol Metab 1998;83:309–19.[5]

patients are high and several-fold higher than the response to GHRH, the latter being normal or often subnormal.[7] GHRH, in addition to GHRP, evokes a synergistic response. The high GH responses to secretagogues credibly exclude a lack of pituitary capacity to *synthesise* GH as the ultimate mechanism underlying the blunted GH secretion during protracted critical illness. This infers that one of the mechanisms involved is a lack of the endogenous ligand(s) for the GHRP receptor. Ultimately, the combination of reduced availability of SRIH and endogenous GHRP-like ligand emerges as a plausible mechanism that clarifies the reduced amplitude of GH pulses, the increased frequency of spontaneous GH secretory bursts and the elevated interpulse levels as well as the striking responsiveness of GHRP alone or in combination with GHRH. This occurs without markedly increased responsiveness to GHRH alone subnormal.[7] Male patients reveal a lower response to GHRP alone than female patients, a difference which is completely abrogated by the addition of GHRH. Less endogenous GHRH action, possibly due to the concomitant profound hypoandrogenism in the men, accompanying loss of the putative endogenous GHRP-like ligand action with prolonged stress in both genders may explain this finding.[6]

The hypothesis of reduced hypothalamic stimulation has been further explored by examining the effects of continuous infusion of GHRH ± GHRP. Continuously infusing GHRP, and even more so GHRH + GHRP, was found to substantially amplify pulsatile GH secretion (> 6-fold and > 10-fold respectively) in this condition, without altering the relatively high burst frequency, an effect that lasted up to 45 hours.[4,8] Reactivated pulsatile GH secretion was accompanied by a proportionate rise in serum IGF-1 by 66% and 106%, IGFBP-3 (50% and 56%) and acid-labile subunit (65% and 97%) indicating peripheral GH responsiveness. The presence of considerable responsiveness to reactivated endogenous GH secretion was verified by a high serum level of GHBP recently documented in this phase and clearly delineates the distinct pathophysiological mechanism of the chronic phase of critical illness, as opposed to the acute phase, which is thought to be primarily a condition of GH resistance. Recent data have shown that the responsiveness to GH secretagogues (co-administered with thyroid-releasing hormone, TRH) in this condition is maintained for at least 5 days, with active feedback inhibition loops preventing overtreatment, restoring (near) normal levels of IGFBPs and evoking an anabolic effect at the level of several peripheral tissues.[5]

Changes in thyroid hormone with critical illness
(Figure 1.4)

The changes within the thyroid axis also have a dual presentation.[9] Within 2 hours after onset of severe physical stress such as for example,

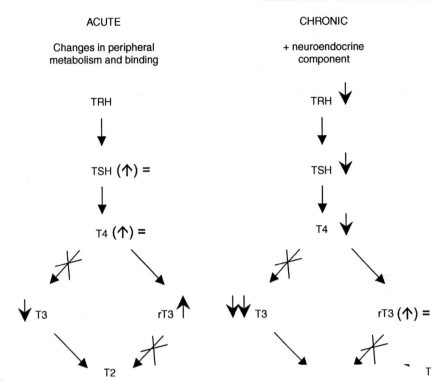

Figure 1.4   A simplified overview of the major changes which occur within the thyroid axis during the acute and chronic phase of critical illness. T2 = diodothyronine; T3 = tri-iodothyronine; rT3 = reverse T3. Reproduced with permission from Van den Berghe G. Eur J Endocrinol 2000 (in press).[9]

surgery, serum levels of triiodothyronine (T3) decrease, whereas thyroxine (T4) and thyroid-stimulating hormone (TSH) briefly rise. Apparently, low T3 levels at that stage are mainly caused by a decreased peripheral conversion of T4 to T3. Subsequently, TSH and T4 levels often return to "normal" whereas T3 levels remain low. The magnitude of the T3 drop within 24 hours has been found to reflect the severity of illness. The cytokines tumour necrosis factor-α (TNF-α), interleukin-1 (IL-1) and IL-6 have been investigated as putative mediators of the acute low T3 syndrome. However, antagonists of these cytokines in sick mice failed to restore normal thyroid function.[10] Low concentrations of binding proteins and inhibition of hormone binding, transport and metabolism by elevated levels of free fatty acids and bilirubin have been proposed as factors contributing to the low T3 syndrome at tissue level. Teleologically, the acute changes in the thyroid axis have been interpreted as an attempt to reduce energy expenditure at least when they occur during starvation, and thus as an appropriate response do not warrant intervention. Where this is

7

also applicable to other acute stress conditions, such as surgery or the initial phase of critical illness, is still not clear.

Patients treated in ICU for weeks or months, however, present with a different set of changes within the thyroid axis.[11] A single sample usually reveals low–normal TSH values for a given assay and low T4 and T3 serum concentrations. However, overnight repeated sampling reveals that, essentially, the pulsatility in the TSH secretory pattern is dramatically diminished and this loss of TSH pulse amplitude is related to low serum levels of T3. Moreover, postmortem examination has shown that after chronic severe illness, TRH mRNA in hypothalamic paraventricular nuclei is reduced whereas this is not the case after death from acute insults. Together, these findings indicate that the reduced production of thyroid hormones in the prolonged phase of critical illness may be caused by impairment of hypothalamic stimulation. In line with this concept is the rise of TSH marking onset of recovery from severe illness.

The neuroendocrine pathogenesis of the low thyroid hormone levels in prolonged critical illness is unknown. As circulating cytokine levels are usually low, other mechanisms operational within the central nervous system are presumably involved. Endogenous dopamine and prolonged hypercortisolism may each play a role; exogenous dopamine is known to provoke or severely aggravate hypothyroidism in critical illness. A recent study has for the first time shown that low thyroid hormone levels in protracted critical illness do not reflect an adaptive, protective mechanism against hypercatabolism since restoring physiological levels of thyroid hormones by continuously infusing TRH (+ GHRP) was found to be associated with a reduction in hypercatabolism.[6] During TRH infusion in prolonged critical illness, the negative feedback exerted by thyroid hormones upon the thyrotropes was found to be maintained, thus precluding overstimulation of the thyroid axis. Moreover, co-infusion of TRH and growth hormone-releasing factors appears a better strategy than TRH alone as this combination seems necessary to also increase the pulsatile fraction of TSH release and to avoid a rise in circulating reverse T3. This finding points to important interaction among different anterior pituitary axes for optimal peripheral responses. In contrast to treatment with thyroid hormones, infusing TRH allows for peripheral shifts in thyroid hormone metabolism during intercurrent events and, accordingly, permits the body to generate appropriate concentrations of thyroid hormones in the circulation and at tissue level, thus setting the scene for a safer treatment than the administration of T3. It remains speculative, however, whether the low serum and tissue concentrations of T3 are also involved in several problems distinctively associated with prolonged critical illness. Outcome benefit of TRH infusion alone or in combination with growth hormone secretagogues in prolonged critical illness is yet to be studied.

Prolactin, luteinizing hormone and adrenocorticotrophin (ACTH)

In line with the observations within the somatotropic and thyroid axes, pulsatile release of prolactin and luteinizing hormone is also impaired in the chronic phase of critical illness. Even the pituitary–adrenal axis responds differently to acute insults and to the chronic stress of protracted critical illness, as evidenced by low circulating levels of adreno-corticotrophin (adrenocorticotrophic hormone, ACTH) in protracted critical illness.

Conclusions

Acute and prolonged critical illness result in different neuroendocrine paradigms which should perhaps be approached with different therapeutic strategies. The acute response to severe illness or trauma consists primarily of an actively secreting anterior pituitary gland and a peripheral inactivation or inactivity of anabolic target organ hormones, a response which is thought to be beneficial and adaptive. In the chronic phase of critical illness, a uniformly reduced pulsatile secretion of anterior pituitary hormones underlies reduced activity of several target tissues. It is unlikely that the reduced hypothalamic stimulation in the chronic phase of illness has been selected by evolution and should accordingly be considered as time-honoured and appropriate. Since infusing the presumed deficient hypothalamic releasing factors respects active feedback-inhibition loops which precludes overtreatment, this approach appears safe in the critically ill. It remains to be determined whether endocrine interventions with releasing factors in prolonged critical illness will accelerate healing and recovery of those patients who need it most.

References

1 Van den Berghe G, de Zegher F, Bouillon R. Acute and prolonged critical illness as different neuroendocrine paradigms. *J Clin Endocrinol Metab* 1998;**83**:1827–34.
2 Kojima M, Hosoda H, Date Y, Nakazato M. Ghrelin is a growth-hormone-releasing acetylated peptide from stomach. *Nature* 1999;**402**:656–60.
3 Hermansson M, Wickelgren RB, Hammerqvist F, *et al.* Measurement of human growth hormone receptor messenger ribonucleic acid by a quantitative polymerase chain reaction-based assay: demonstration of reduced expression after elective surgery. *J Clin Endocrinol Metab* 1997;**82**:421–8.

4 Van den Berghe G, de Zegher F, Baxter RC, *et al.* Neuroendocrinology of prolonged critical illness: effect of continuous thyrotropin-releasing hormone infusion and its combination with growth hormone-secretagogues. *J Clin Endocrinol Metab* 1998;**83**:309–19.

5 Van den Berghe G, Wouters P, Weekers F, *et al.* Reactivation of pituitary hormone release and metabolic improvement by infusion of growth hormone releasing peptide and thyrotropin-releasing hormone in patients with protracted critical illness. *J Clin Endocrinol Metab* 1999;**84**:1311–23.

6 Van den Berghe G, Baxter RC, Weekers F, *et al.* A paradoxical gender dissociation within the growth hormone/insulin-like growth factor 1 axis during protracted critical illness. *J Clin Endocrinol Metab* 2000;**85**:183–92.

7 Van den Berghe G, de Zegher F, Bowers C, *et al.* Pituitary responsiveness to growth hormone (GH) releasing hormone, GH-releasing peptide-2 and thyrotropin releasing hormone in critical illness. *Clin Endocrinol* 1996;**45**;341–51.

8 Van den Berghe G, de Zegher F, Veldhuis JD, *et al.* The somatotropic axis in critical illness: effect of continuous GHRH and GHRP-2 infusion. *J Clin Endocrinol Metab* 1997;**82**:590–9.

9 Van den Berghe G. Novel insights in the neuroendocrinology of critical illness. *Eur J Endocrinol* 2000 (in press).

10 van der Poll T, van Zee K, Endert E, *et al.* Interleukin-1 receptor blockade does not affect endotoxin-induced changes in plasma thyroid hormone and thyrotropin concentration in man. *J Clin Endocrinol Metab* 1995;**80**:1341–6

11 Van den Berghe G, de Zegher F, Veldhuis JD, *et al.* Thyrotropin and prolactin release in prolonged critical illness: dynamics of spontaneous secretion and effects of growth hormone secretagogues. *Clin Endocrinol* 1997;**47**:599–612.

2: Growth hormone therapy in the critically ill

CHARLES HINDS

Introduction

Complex alterations in the growth hormone/insulin-like growth factor (GH/IGF) axis are thought to play an important role in the protein catabolism which complicates trauma, burns, sepsis and major surgical procedures. Although basal GH levels are sometimes increased, oscillatory activity is frequently attenuated and in prolonged critical illness blunted GH secretion has been shown to consist of a large number of small secretory bursts superimposed on basal release, in part due to changes in the hypothalamus.[1] This reduction in pulsatile GH secretion, probably combined, at least in the early stages, with GH resistance contributes to the fall in circulating levels of IGF-1 and its major binding protein IGFBP-3 which has been described consistently in the critically ill.[2] As a result of these changes the indirect anabolic actions of GH mediated by IGF-1 are reduced, whilst in the acute phase, raised basal GH levels lead to increased lipolysis and insulin antagonism. The fall in circulating IGF-1 promotes muscle catabolism, yielding amino acids such as glutamine for protein synthesis in rapidly dividing cells (e.g. gut mucosa and leucocytes) and for wound healing, whilst avoiding the hazards of hypoglycaemia. These adaptive changes may be of benefit in the short term but in the context of modern intensive care, where seriously ill patients often survive for many days or weeks and nutritional support is available, they can lead to severe muscle wasting and weakness, which may prolong weaning from mechanical ventilation and delay mobilisation, as well as compromising tissue repair, wound healing and immune function. Not surprisingly, the magnitude of protein loss is closely related to a poor outcome and such patients consume a disproportionate share of resources.

There are now a large number of studies demonstrating that the administration of high doses of recombinant human growth hormone (5–20-fold the dose needed for replacement therapy in GH-deficient adults) can improve nitrogen balance in normal subjects receiving hypocaloric parenteral

11

nutrition, patients with severe burns, patients with trauma receiving parenteral nutrition, patients who have undergone surgery, patients in the early phase of sepsis, and other categories of critically ill patient. There is, however, only limited evidence that the reduction in nitrogen losses translates into clinically important functional benefits or improvements in outcome. Although it has been suggested that GH can facilitate weaning from mechanical ventilation, in one relatively small, prospective, randomised controlled study, treatment with GH was not associated with preservation of muscle strength or a shortened period of weaning, despite marked nitrogen retention.[3] On the other hand, this, and a number of other relatively small studies, have indicated that treatment with supraphysiological doses of GH is safe in patients with sepsis, and severe sepsis, as well as in critically ill patients without sepsis. Moreover, in seriously ill postoperative patients with respiratory failure given high doses of GH, the mortality rate was lower than predicted[4] and in one retrospective study GH treatment was associated with increased survival of adults with severe burns.[5] It therefore came as a considerable surprise when two prospective, randomised, controlled trials demonstrated that administration of recombinant human GH (rhGH) to long stay critically ill adults during the first few weeks of the acute illness was associated with a significant increase in mortality, as well as prolongation of weaning times, duration of intensive care and length of hospital stay.[6]

Were we right to give growth hormone in the first place?

Although we embarked on this study with an entirely open mind it never occurred to the participating clinicians that mortality might actually be increased by GH treatment. Of course there will always be those who say with hindsight, "Well, I never thought it would work, I don't know why you bothered," and there are even some who will say "I knew it was going to be dangerous." Of course one knows that if a smaller dose had failed to have an effect, the enthusiasts would have said "If you had used a bigger dose you would have shown benefit." Others have suggested that the wrong sort of patients were treated or that they were treated either too early or too late. Another obvious criticism is that the trial involved heterogeneous groups of patients. There are also a number of legitimate questions concerning the rationale behind the study, the conduct of the study and the design of the study. The remainder of this article will address these issues.

Rationale for administering growth hormone to critically ill patients

Giving huge doses of growth hormone to extremely sick, ventilated patients on the intensive care unit (ICU) may seem strange to those who are not particularly familiar with the field. So why did we do it? We know that extensive surgery, trauma and sepsis are complicated by a catabolic response, which is characterised by a number of well-known metabolic changes, including a negative nitrogen balance. We are all too well aware that this can cause for example, impaired wound healing, delayed tissue repair and immunosuppression. Muscle wasting can delay mobilisation and weaning from the ventilator and these in turn may prolong ICU and hospital stay (see above). For this reason, it seemed to be entirely reasonable to attempt to either prevent or limit this catabolic response, although in the light of our findings, some have suggested that we should revisit even this most basic of premises.

It is thought that the protein loss which complicates critical illness is a consequence of a disturbed GH/IGF axis. This is interpreted conventionally as a state of growth hormone resistance and provides the rational for administering supraphysiological doses of growth hormone in an attempt to improve nitrogen balance in catabolic patients. But the situation is probably rather more complex than this and certainly more so than was appreciated when the growth hormone study was designed.

What was the evidence that growth hormone therapy might work?

Given the central role of IGF in mediating the anabolic effects of growth hormone, one would anticipate that in order for growth hormone to be effective its administration would have to be associated with increases in circulating levels of IGF. Certainly this seems to be the case. In burns patients for example, administration of growth hormone is associated with significant increases in circulating levels of IGF, although it is worth noting that this increase in IGF is less impressive in the more severely burned patients.

In patients who had undergone open cholecystectomy and were receiving total parenteral nutrition (TPN), growth hormone administration significantly improved postoperative nitrogen balance.[7] Even when given early after ICU admission to patients with severe sepsis, an improvement in nitrogen balance was seen, although this was, admittedly, rather modest. Importantly, because muscle protein synthesis is closely related to muscle glutamine levels, the improvement in nitrogen balance achieved with growth hormone is associated with a reduction in the extent of the postoperative decrease in muscle glutamine levels.

There is, however, only limited evidence that these potentially beneficial effects of growth hormone on nitrogen economy are associated with either functional improvements or improvements in clinically relevant endpoints. Certainly, growth hormone administration to postoperative patients has been associated with an improvement in hand grip strength and subjective improvements in the ability to cough.

Why did we think it would be safe?

In a relatively small study of growth hormone administration in critically ill but non septic patients there was no suggestion that mortality was increased by growth hormone.[8] Similarly, in another relatively small study from the same group, there was again no suggestion of increased mortality.[9] Perhaps most importantly, in a study of patients with severe sepsis from the same group, there was no suggestion that mortality was increased, with only two deaths in the growth hormone group and three in the control group.[10] Finally, in a study of surgical patients with sepsis, although one patient in the growth hormone group did die, there was no indication of increased mortality.[11] In none of these studies did growth hormone administration seem to be associated with any side effects or adverse events.

Why did we need to perform another trial?

One might ask, therefore why was it necessary to perform another trial? Well, of course, some previous studies were limited by small numbers, some by being retrospective and some by not being randomised. Moreover, findings have been conflicting and growth hormone does not consistently improve nitrogen balance in the more seriously ill patients. In a study of immobilised, severely traumatised patients, for example, growth hormone failed to improve nitrogen balance.[12] It was also unclear whether growth hormone treatment could produce clinically important functional improvements; for example, in the study by Pichard et al.,[3] growth hormone administration improved nitrogen balance but failed to reduce the cumulative mechanical ventilation time. On the other hand, in a retrospective study there was some suggestion that growth hormone treatment could actually improve survival rates in patients with burns.[5] In this latter study, the authors retrospectively divided patients into those who had received growth hormone and those who had not. The patients given growth hormone had a mortality rate of 11% whilst 37% of those who had not received growth hormone died, despite the fact that the growth hormone recipients were rather more seriously ill. In another study from the same group, patients with postoperative respiratory failure were given growth hormone. This was not a randomised study, but the mortality rate in the growth hormone treated patients was significantly lower than would have been predicted.[4] Thus there was sufficient uncertainty to warrant a prospective randomised controlled trial, in particular to determine whether growth hormone administration could lead to improvement in clinically important outcome measures in critically ill adults.

The trials

Two prospective, randomised controlled studies evaluating the effects of administering recombinant human growth hormone to long-stay critically ill adults were conducted independently, but in parallel.[6] The Finnish study was performed in six hospitals in Finland, and the European study in a number of ICUs elsewhere in Europe. The duration of ICU stay was the primary efficacy variable. Secondary efficacy variables included utilisation of ICU resources assessed by the therapeutic intervention scoring system (TISS), time on the ventilator, and time in hospital. Hand grip strength, exercise tolerance, organ failures and nitrogen balance (in the Finnish study) were also determined. Hospital mortality was recorded. Patients were eligible for recruitment if they were 18–80 years old and had been on the ICU for 5–7 days and were expected to remain for at least another 5 days. For safety reasons there were a large number of exclusion criteria, including insulin-dependent diabetes, liver dysfunction and malignancy. Because efficacy had previously been shown in patients with burns, these patients were excluded from the study, and for obvious reasons we excluded patients with pre-existing neuromuscular disorders. Severity of illness was assessed using the APACHE II score, on admission and every 3 days thereafter. Routine haematology and biochemistry were recorded, and circulating levels of IGF-1 and the binding protein IGFBP-3 were determined. Daily vital signs were recorded. Adverse events and overall mortality were continuously monitored throughout the study, but by a safety committee blinded to treatment groups.

In both studies, patients in the growth hormone and placebo groups were similar in terms of sex distribution, age, body weight, although the Finnish patients were slightly heavier than the European patients. The distribution between the diagnostic groups (respiratory failure, postcardiac surgery, abdominal surgery, trauma) was also similar. Energy intake was similar between studies and between groups. Nitrogen balance was slightly higher in the Finnish patients, but the dose of growth hormone was identical. Not surprisingly, administration of growth hormone was associated with a significant increase in insulin requirements, although blood glucose levels were fairly well controlled by the higher doses of insulin. As expected, growth hormone administration was associated with significant increases in circulating levels of IGF-1 and IGFBP-3. In the Finnish study, growth hormone administration was associated with an improvement in nitrogen balance.

Mortality

On completion of the Finnish study, mortality was checked. Unexpectedly, the mortality in the growth hormone group was around 40% and in the placebo group approximately 20%. In the multinational study, there was a very similar, highly significant increase in mortality in the growth hormone group. This increased mortality was consistent throughout all the four diagnostic groups and all the APACHE score bands (Table 2.1), and persisted for up to six months. Not only was mortality increased, but there was also evidence that growth hormone increased morbidity. The duration of mechanical ventilation was longer in the growth hormone group, as was the duration of ICU and hospital stay. There was no effect of growth hormone on hand grip strength or exercise tolerance. Two independent physicians who were blinded to the study group allocation assessed the causes of death in all non-survivors. Not surprisingly, the commonest cause of death was multiple-organ failure and septic shock but this predominance was most obvious in the GH group. It is also worth noting that sepsis was reported as an adverse event much more frequently in the growth hormone-treated patients.

The lessons

Despite innumerable meetings and discussions the reason(s) for the increased morbidity and mortality associated with growth hormone treatment in these studies remains unclear. Nevertheless, the preponderance of multiple-organ failure and septic shock or uncontrolled infection as causes of death in the growth hormone group suggests that modulation of immune function might have been involved. Another possible explanation is that rhGH prevented the mobilisation of glutamine from muscle and that, as a result, less glutamine was available for rapidly dividing cells, such as leucocytes and enterocytes, and for hepatic production of glutathione. Other suggestions have included fluid retention, insulin resistance, stimulation of lipolysis, and interference with thyroid or adrenocortical function. In some cases these side effects may have been amplified by concomitant endocrine deficiencies such as hypothyroidism and adrenal insufficiency. The deleterious effects of growth hormone in critically ill patients are probably multifactorial, complex, interlinked, and dependent on the timing of treatment, the patient's condition and the dose of growth hormone. Further investigations are therefore required to determine the mechanism(s) underlying these adverse effects of GH.

It can be categorically concluded, however, that giving high doses of growth hormone to long-stay critically ill adults, at least during the first few

Table 2.1 In-hospital deaths and causes of death during intensive care

Deaths and causes	Finnish study			Multinational study		
	Growth hormone (n = 119)	Placebo (n = 123)	p value	Growth hormone (n = 139)	Placebo (n = 141)	p value
Deaths						
Total number of patients (%)	47 (39)	25 (20)	< 0.001	61 (44)	26 (18)	< 0.001
Relative risk of death (95% CI)	1.9 (1.3–2.9)			2.4 (1.6–3.5)		
Diagnostic group: number of patients/total number (%)						
Cardiac surgery	10/24 (42)	6/25 (24)		21/40 (52)	8/47 (17)	
Abdominal surgery	17/33 (52)	11/36 (31)		12/25 (48)	10/25 (40)	
Trauma	2/7 (29)	1/8 (12)		4/20 (20)	1/25 (4)	
Acute respiratory failure	18/55 (33)	7/54 (13)		24/54 (44)	7/44 (16)	
APACHE II score during first 24 h: number of patients/total number (%)						
≤ 20	30/79 (38)	12/83 (14)		42/100 (42)	13/92 (14)	
> 20	17/40 (42)	13/40 (32)		19/39 (49)	13/49 (27)	
APACHE II score at enrollment: number of patients/total number (%)						
≤ 20	34/97 (35)	22/110 (20)		43/115 (37)	16/115 (14)	
> 20	13/22 (59)	3/13 (23)		18/24 (75)	10/26 (38)	
Age: number of patients/total number (%)						
< 55 years	9/36 (25)	7/47 (15)		8/34 (24)	0/35	
55–70 years	17/45 (38)	7/44 (16)		28/61 (46)	14/61 (23)	
> 70 years	21/38 (55)	11/32 (34)		25/44 (57)	12/45 (27)	
Causes of death during intensive care: number of patients			0.66			0.71
Multiple-organ failure	12	6		22	11	
Septic shock or uncontrolled infection	15	4		16	4	
Cardiovascular cause	3	2		9	2	
Refractory respiratory failure	2	1		4	1	
Other	4	4		3	2	

* p values are comparisons between treatment groups in each study.   CI = confidence interval. APACHE = Acute physiology and chronic health evaluation score.

Reproduced and adapted with permission from Takala J, Ruokonen E, Webster NR, et al. N Engl J Med 1999;**341**:785–92.[6]

weeks of their illness, is associated with increased morbidity and mortality. Given that there are over ninety publications in the literature since the mid-1950s in which growth hormone has been administered to catabolic patients without any suggestion of adverse effects, this unexpected finding emphasises the importance of continuing to perform prospective randomised controlled trials in critically ill patients, despite the difficulties inherent in designing, conducting and interpreting such studies. Conducting independent parallel studies may provide a useful model for trials in the future, since in this way any suggestion that the results are a chance finding can be refuted. It is also clear that all randomised studies in intensive care patients should involve an unblinded safety committee.

References

1 Van den Berghe G, De Zegher F, Veldhuis JD, *et al*. The somatotropic axis in critical illness: effect of continuous growth hormone (GH)-releasing hormone and GH-releasing peptide-2 infusion. *J Clin Endocrinol Metab* 1997;**82:**590–9.

2 Timmins AC, Cotterill AM, Hughes SC, *et al*. Critical illness is associated with low circulating concentrations of insulin-like growth factors-I and –II, alterations in insulin-like growth factor binding proteins, and induction of insulin-like growth factor binding protein 3 protease. *Crit Care Med* 1996;**24:**1460–6.

3 Pichard C, Kyle U, Chevrolet J-C, *et al*. Lack of effects of recombinant growth hormone on muscle function in patients requiring prolonged mechanical ventilation: a prospective, randomized, controlled study. *Crit Care Med* 1996;**24:**403–13.

4 Knox JB, Wilmore DW, Demling RH, *et al*. Use of growth hormone for postoperative respiratory failure. *Am J Surg* 1996;**171:**576–80.

5 Knox J, Demling R, Wilmore D, *et al*. Increased survival after major thermal injury: the effect of growth hormone therapy in adults. *J Trauma* 1995;**39:**526–30.

6 Takala J, Ruokonen E, Webster NR, *et al*. Increased mortality associated with growth hormone treatment in critically ill adults. *N Engl J Med* 1999;**341:**785–92.

7 Harmqvist F, Stromberg C, von der Decken A, *et al*. Biosynthetic human growth hormone preserves both muscle protein synthesis and the decrease in muscle-free glutamine, and improves whole-body nitrogen economy after operation. *Ann Surg* 1992;**216:**184–91.

8 Voermann BJ, Strack van Schijndel RJM, Groeneveld ABJ, *et al*. Effects of human growth hormone in critically ill non-septic patients: results from a prospective, randomised, placebo-controlled trial. *Crit Care Med* 1995;**23:**665–73.

9 Voerman BJ, Strack van Schijndel RJ, de Boer H, *et al*. Effects of human growth hormone on fuel utilisation and mineral balance in critically ill patients on full intravenous nutritional support. *J Crit Care* 1994;**9:**143–50.

10 Voerman BJ, Schijndel RJM, Groeneveld ABJ, *et al*. Effects of recombinant human growth hormone in patients with severe sepsis. *Ann Surg* 1992;**216:**648–55.

11 Koea JB, Breier BH, Douglas RG, *et al.* Anabolic and cardiovascular effects of recombinant human growth hormone in surgical patients with sepsis. *Br J Surg* 1996;**83**:196–202.
12 Behrman SW, Kudsk KA, Brown RO, *et al.* The effect of GH on nutritional markers in enterally fed immobilised trauma patients. *J Parent Ent Nutr* 1995;**19**:41–6.

3: Thyroid disturbance in the critically ill

ANTHONY P WEETMAN

Introduction

Thyroid disturbance in the critically ill covers both the non-specific disturbances in many sick patients that can lead to abnormality in conventional thyroid function tests. These may confuse the unwary, since flu's situation is referred to as sick euthyroid syndrome which presupposes that these patients are truly euthyroid, although this supposition has been challenged. Also, the true but rare, thyroid emergencies of thyrotoxicosis crisis and myxoedema coma will be discussed.

Sick euthyroid syndrome

Any acute, severe illness can cause abnormalities of circulating thyroid-stimulating hormone (TSH) or thyroid hormone levels in the absence of thyroid disease, making these measurements potentially misleading.[1,2] It follows that, unless a thyroid disorder is strongly suspected, there is no place for "routine" testing of thyroid function in sick patients. The real hallmark of the sick euthyroid syndrome is that the changes in thyroid hormone levels are reversed with recovery from the precipitating illness. If the patient truly has a thyroid illness these non-specific effects may obscure the features of that thyroid illness. Indeed there are cases of normal thyroid hormone levels in patients who in reality are thyrotoxic, but severe acute illness has caused such profound effects that thyroid hormone levels are normal.

The basic pathway for thyroid hormone metabolism is shown in Figure 3.1. Thyroxine (T4) is an inactive hormone which has no effect on the cell; for biological activity it has to be converted to tri-iodothyronine (T3). Most of T3 which is actually active at the cellular level is derived from peripheral conversion rather than thyroidal secretion. This conversion is dependent primarily on type 1 deiodinase, which is found predoinantly in the liver, the

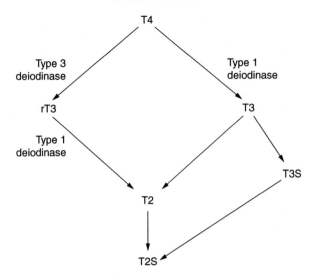

Figure 3.1 Simplified metabolic pathway of thyroid hormones. T2 = diodothyronine; T3 = triodothyronine; rT3 = reverse T3; T2S = sulphated T2; T3S = sulphated T3.

main site of T3 conversion in the body. There is another pathway to T4 conversion, mediated by type 3 deiodinase which converts T4 to reverse T3, which is totally biologically inactive. Type 1 deiodinase in the liver then converts reverse T3 to diiodothyronine (T2) (Figure 3.1). For simplicity, type 2 deiodinase is missing from Figure 3.1. This is an enzyme which is particularly found in the pituitary and is responsible for ensuring the pituitary gets its own supply of T3.

During illness, the most common pattern of change of thyroid hormones is a decrease in total and free T3 levels with normal levels of T4 and TSH. The magnitude of the fall in T3 correlates with the severity of the illness. T4 conversion to T3 via hepatic deiodination is impaired and there is a rise in reverse T3 (rT3) but this is due to decreased clearance rather than increased production; it is likely that T4 is alternatively metabolised to the hormonally inactive T3 sulphate. This low T3 state can be induced rapidly even by fasting in normal subjects, and may be a mechanism to limit gluconeogenesis from muscle. Thus, the low T3 state may limit catabolism in ill patients, and it is generally assumed that it requires no treatment. However, this view has recently been questioned.[3]

Very ill patients may have a fall in total T4 as well as in T3 levels, due to altered binding to serum proteins, and this state has a poor prognosis which is not altered by thyroid hormone administration. Modern free T4 assays usually give a normal free T4 level in such patients depending on the method used: some assays produce values which are subnormal or even

21

raised in this setting. TSH levels in sick patients can also be raised or lowered and values of <0.1 or >20 mU/L occur in 2–3% of cases, levels which are otherwise strongly suggestive of thyrotoxicosis or hypothyroidism. Dopamine, a rise in endogenous cortisol, or administration of glucocorticoids, provides a partial explanation for the decrease in TSH levels, and cytokines may also be involved. However, the exact mechanisms underlying the subnormal TSH seen in 10% of sick patients, and the rise in TSH level seen in 5%, remains unclear.

It is important to note that some of the reported changes in thyroid hormone levels, but by no means all, are determined by the type of assay which is used to measure thyroid hormone. Therefore, each laboratory, using a particular type of assay, may find a consistent trend in one direction, particularly for free thyroid hormone levels. However, a different laboratory using a different type of assay may produce different values.

The sick euthyroid syndrome can occur in any setting of severe illness, including severe infection, major surgery, myocardial infarction, starvation, liver disease and kidney disease. The cause of these changes, which occur for any type of illness, is unknown. Reduced hepatic uptake and metabolism of T4 is one important factor, although the mechanism is obscure, and release of cytokines is also involved. Drugs can also be responsible for some of the changes; in particular, dopamine can affect TSH, leading to a fall in TSH. Glucocorticoids, particularly in high doses, can suppress TSH levels and at the same time very high doses of glucocorticoids can interfere with thyroid hormone metabolism. Of course, it is the use of these drugs which is not always accounted for in studies, that add a further layer of complexity to interpretation of thyroid hormone changes.

Mortality correlates with the severity of the thyroid hormone changes. In patients with no change, mortality was 0.8% and length of hospital stay 8 days in one large series.[1] In a second group, who had a rise in rT3, there was a 10-fold increase in mortality and twice the length of stay in hospital. At the next degree of severity, where rT3 was raised but T3 levels declined, mortality was increased 3-fold and length of stay was further increased. The most profound changes occurred in the most severely ill group, with the highest mortality and the longest length of stay. In this high mortality group, there was a fall in both T3 and T4 levels. These data strongly suggest that the more severe the thyroid hormone changes the more likely the patient is to have an adverse outcome.[1]

What causes the low T3 and the raised rT3? Physiology suggests that the obvious explanation for this would be an impairment in type 1 deiodination. However, the most important cause is a reduced T4 and rT3 uptake into hepatocytes. This would result in low T3 and raised rT3 levels. There is no in vitro evidence for impairment of type 1 deiodinase activity. Thus it is not deiodinase activity itself which is impaired but impaired uptake of T4 and rT3 which accounts for the bulk of these changes.

What about the fall in T4? T4 can be measured in two ways; as total T4 level or free T4 level. There is no doubt that any fall in total T4 level is due to a fall in thyroxine binding globulin (TBG), the major binding hormone for T4. This occurs particularly in those patients with liver and renal disease. In the vast majority of patients the fall in total T4 is due to reduction in TBG concentration. Changes in free T4 are the most difficult to understand. At least some of these changes are assay dependent and it may well be that in some assays there is inhibited hormone binding due to the presence of inhibitors. These inhibitors may displace thyroid hormones from their binding protein, thereby raising levels. As mentioned above there is also reduced hepatic uptake of free T4 which may tend to raise free T4 levels. Tumour necrosis factor (TNF-α) can cause a rise in free T4 levels. However, the overall effect on thyroid hormone levels that we now realise is most important in those patients with high mortality comes about through changes in TSH. TSH alterations are independent of any changes in circulating T3 and T4 in sick euthyroid syndrome, suggesting a defect at the hypothalamic level.

Even when dopamine and glucocorticoid administration have been excluded as a cause of reduced TSH, such changes are still seen in many patients with acute illness. It now seems fairly clear that cytokines are involved in these non-drug associated cases. The two cytokines which seem to be of major importance are tumour necrosis factor-α (TNF-α) and interleukin-6 (IL-6) with a possible role for IL-1. However, there may well be other cytokines or inflammatory mediators which independently act on the hypothalamus and the pituitary. Even in very sick people, TSH values fall to a level compatible with levels which occur in patients with overt thyrotoxicosis, such that TSH levels cannot discriminate between true thyrotoxicosis and non-thyroidal illness, even with the most sensitive TSH assay. However, the lower the TSH the more likely the patient is to be thyrotoxic.

Although any severe illness or trauma can induce changes in thyroid hormone levels, certain disorders give a distinctive pattern of abnormalities. Acute liver disease is associated with an initial rise in total (but not free) T3 and T4 levels, due to thyroxine binding globulin release; these levels become subnormal with progression to liver failure. A transient increase in total and free T4 levels, usually with a normal T3 level, is found in 5–30% of acutely ill psychiatric patients. TSH values may be low, normal or high, and all abnormalities tend to revert to normal 1–2 weeks after hospitalisation. In the early stage of human immunodeficiency virus (HIV) infection T3 and T4 levels rise, even if there is weight loss, but T3 then falls with progression to acquired immune deficiency syndrome (AIDS); TSH levels usually remain normal. Renal disease is often accompanied by low T3 concentrations, but with normal rather than raised rT3 levels, due to an unknown factor increasing uptake of rT3 into the liver.

23

The question remains as to whether the sick thyroid syndrome should be treated. Conventional dogma is that some of these changes are due to inhibitors which do not affect the situation at the tissue level. However, some studies have shown that tissue thyroid hormone content is truly low, but this may represent a physiological response which is not harmful. There have been no adequate studies in man to try and address this question. Most studies previously have used therapeutic administration of T4, but impaired T4 uptake occurs in illness, such that this approach would not adequately treat a low thyroid state. Therefore one would need to give T3 intravenously, ideally together with T4 in order to achieve tissue saturation with thyroid hormone, if the patient really was hypothyroid at the tissue level. Of course, there are concerns about administration of T3 and the effect of treatment on the heart. Although a randomised controlled trial is needed, such a study would be quite daunting, since to detect a 20% improvement in a 20% mortality group at significant levels, 1500 patients would need to be studied.

Myxoedema coma

Myxoedema coma (Box 3.1) occurs particularly in newly diagnosed or poorly controlled patients and is almost unheard of in patients below the age of 60. Despite intensive treatment, this condition has a mortality rate of around 50%. Patients present with features of hypothyroidism, unconsciousness or seizures, and hypothermia which can reach as low as 23°C. There may be a history of poor compliance with T4 treatment, or the patient may be previously undiagnosed. Myxoedema coma is precipitated by factors which impair respiration, especially drugs, pneumonia, congestive heart failure, myocardial infarction, gastrointestinal bleeding or stroke. Exposure to cold may also be a risk factor. Hypoventilation, causing hypoxia and hypercapnia, plays a major role in the development of coma but hypoglycaemia and dilutional hyponatraemia also contribute.

Myxoedema coma should be treated vigorously when suspected, with-

---

Box 3.1   Characteristics of myxoedema coma

- Hypothyroidism
- Profound hypothermia
- Coma, seizures
- 50% mortality

---

out awaiting biochemical confirmation. Treatment consists of thyroid hormone replacement, supportive measures and treatment of any underlying precipitant. No method of thyroid hormone replacement has proven superiority.[4] Thyroxine can be given as a single intravenous bolus of 500 µg; although further replacement is not strictly necessary for several days, it is often given at the usual dose of 50–100 µg/day after a bolus. If a suitable intravenous preparation is unavailable, the same initial dose of thyroxine can be given by nasogastric tube (but absorption may be impaired). An alternative is to give triiodothyronine, intravenously or via nasogastric tube, in doses ranging from 10 µg every 4–6 hours to 25 µg every 12 hours. This treatment has been advocated because T4 to T3 conversion can be impaired in myxoedema coma but it has the potential to provoke arrhythmias. A further variation is to combine thyroxine (200 µg) and triiodothyronine (25 µg) as a single, initial intravenous or oral bolus.

External warming is indicated only if the temperature is below 30°C as it can otherwise cause cardiovascular collapse. Space blankets prevent further heat loss. Parenteral hydrocortisone (50 mg every 6 hours) should be given as there is impaired adrenal reserve in profound hypothyroidism. Early use of broad-spectrum antibiotics, pending the exclusion of infection as a cause is recommended. Ventilatory support is usually needed during the first 48 hours. Hyponatraemia or hypoglycaemia may need correction. Hypotonic intravenous fluids should be avoided as these may exacerbate the water retention secondary to inappropriate vasopressin secretion and reduced renal perfusion.

Thyrotoxic crisis

Thyrotoxic crisis (or thyroid storm; Box 3.2) is rare and presents as a life-threatening exacerbation of hyperthyroidism, accompanied by marked fever, seizures, coma, vomiting, diarrhoea or jaundice.[5] The mortality (due

---

Box 3.2 Characteristics of thyrotoxic crisis

● Severe hyperthyroidism
● Fever
● Seizures, coma
● Vomiting, diarrhoea or jaundice
● Mortality 30% with treatment

---

to cardiac failure, arrhythmia or hyperthermia) is around 30% with treatment and inevitable without. Thyrotoxic crisis is usually precipitated in a patient with partially treated or untreated hyperthyroidism by acute illness (e.g. stroke, infection, trauma, diabetic ketoacidosis), surgery (especially on the thyroid) or radioiodine. Treatment requires close monitoring and consists of measures to reduce thyroid hormone synthesis, supportive therapy, and identification and treatment of the precipitating cause.

Large doses of propylthiouracil (500 mg loading dose and 250 mg 6 hourly) should be given by stomach tube or per rectum. One hour after the first dose of propylthiouracil, stable iodine is given to block thyroid hormone synthesis and release. A saturated solution of potassium iodide (Lugol's iodine), 5 drops every 6 hours, or ipodate 500 mg every 12 hours may be given orally. Sodium iodide 0.25 g intravenously every 6 hours is an alternative but not generally available. Propranolol is also given orally (40–80 mg 4 hourly) or intravenously 2 mg 4 hourly). Caution is needed with heart failure, but controlling the heart rate is crucial in reversing failure in many patients. Supportive measures include glucocorticoids, such as dexamethasone, 2 mg every 6 hours, cooling and intravenous fluids.

There are no clear diagnostic criteria and measurement of thyroid hormone levels are not considered to be useful. Scoring systems have been developed which award points for the severity of fever, central nervous system manifestations, tachycardia and cardiac failure in an attempt to identify the most severely ill patients. Why patients should suddenly go from a fairly stable thyrotoxic state into a crisis is really unknown. It is thought that perhaps there may be saturation of hormone binding sites but no hard data are available to confirm that.

References

1 Docter R, Krenning EP, de Jong M, Hennermann G. The sick euthyroid syndrome: changes in thyroid hormone serum parameters and hormone metabolism. *Clin Endocrinol* 1993;**39**:499–518.
2 McIver B, Gorman CA. Euthyroid sick syndrome: an overview. *Thyroid* 1997;**7**:125–32.
3 De Groot LJ. Dangerous dogmas in medicine: the nonthyroidal illness syndrome. *J Clin Endocrinol Metab* 1999;**84**:151–64.
4 Roti E, Minelli R, Gardini E, Braverman LE. The use and misuse of thyroid hormone. *Endocrine Rev* 1993;**14**:401–23.
5 Burch HB, Wartofsky L. Life-threatening thyrotoxicosis. *Endo Metab Clin N Am* 1993;**22**:263–77.

4: Diabetes for the intensivist

K GEORGE ALBERTI

Introduction

This article will provide an overview of diabetes particularly in relation to those involved in the care of the critically ill. Classification, diagnosis, risk factors, routine and emergency management of patients with diabetes will be addressed.

Classification

Classification of diabetes is important since this has changed recently, to avoid confusion with the overlapping terms insulin and non-insulin-dependent diabetes (Table 4.1). Now we have just type 1 and type 2 diabetes;[1] Type 1 includes classical juvenile-onset autoimmune diabetes although it can also occur in the elderly. Type 1 diabetes involves β-cell destruction, and is mainly an autoimmune condition, although in some patients, particularly those from ethnic minorities, autoantibodies cannot

Table 4.1 Classification of diabetes

New classification	Characteristic	Previous nomenclature
Type 1		Insulin-dependent diabetes
	Mainly autoimmune mechanism	Juvenile onset diabetes
Type 2	Insulin resistant	Non-insulin-dependent diabetes
	Insulin hyposecretion	Maturity-onset diabetes
Gestational		
Other specific types	Genetic disorders	MODY
	Secondary to endocrinopathies, drugs etc.	Secondary diabetes, MRDM

MODY = Mature onset diabetes of the young.
MRDM = Malnutrition related diabetes mellitus.

be demonstrated. Type 2 diabetes includes most other types of diabetes, characterised by insulin hyposecretion and insulin resistance. "Other specific types" includes maturity-onset diabetes of the young, which is a group of genetically based disorders, while the final category is gestational diabetes. The other notable change is that the different stages of the disease can be addressed within the same classification. In type 1 diabetes, for example, if autoantibodies are already present, despite being normoglycaemic, the type 1 classification still holds, however a patient can also be type 1 with a requirement for insulin for survival. In the type 2 classification, a grossly overweight patient can lose 50 kg, which is unlikely, but occasionally happens, normoglycaemia will follow, yet the type 2 process continues. In the intensive care unit (ICU) patients are generally type 2 although they will usually require insulin treatment.

Diagnosis

The criteria for the diagnosis of diabetes have also changed since the diagnostic level of fasting plasma glucose was set in 1979. This is now thought to be too high. The new diagnostic categories[1] are shown in Table 4.2. A new idea which is gaining credence is that a fasting glucose concentration above normal, but not diabetic, suggests that the risk of developing diabetes over the next 5–10 years is likely to be 30%. Similarly, impaired glucose tolerance, defined as a fasting plasma glucose level of less than 7 mmol/L but a 2-hour postglucose load value of 7.8–11 mmol/L suggests the potential for problems in the future.

Table 4.2 Diagnostic criteria for diabetes

- Symptoms + casual plasma glucose ≥ 11 mmol/L
  or
  fasting plasma glucose ≥ 7 mmol/L
  or
  2-h plasma glucose in oral glucose tolerance test ≥ 11 mol/L

- Other abnormalities
  1. Impaired fasting plasma glucose: 6.1–6.9 mmol/L
  2. Impaired glucose tolerance: fasting plasma glucose <7 mmol/L and 2-h plasma glucose after oral glucose tolerance test 7.8–11 mmol/L

Prevalence and risk

Diabetes is not an uncommon disorder. Table 4.3 shows the projected prevalence of diabetes world wide. It can be seen that in 1994, 110 million

Table 4.3 Worldwide prevalence of diabetes

Type	Actual (millions)	Projected (millions)	
	1994	2000	2010
Type 1	11	18	24
Type 2	99	157	215
Total	110	175	239

Table 4.4 The effect of age on diabetes risk

	Age	
Gender	60–69 years	70–79 years
Male	12.8%	19.8%
Female	12.7%	31.4%

people had diabetes; in 2000 the projected figure is 175 million.[2] This is already an underestimate; in the United Kingdom the figure has moved from 2 or 3% up to more than 4% in adults. The risk factors for type 2 diabetes are listed in Box 4.1. The most obvious of course is age. In the over 70s it can be seen that one-third of females have diabetes and 20% of males have diabetes,[3] shown in Table 4.4. It is estimated that this older age group will triple in numbers in the next 15–20 years, so that many more patients will fall into this category, resulting in many more people with diabetes. Another major risk factor is family history. If someone has a first-degree relative with non-insulin type 2 diabetes, they have a 40% lifetime chance of developing diabetes themselves and this risk increases to 50% if there are

---

Box 4.1   Risk factors for type 2 diabetes

- Age
- Family history
- Ethnic origin
- Obesity (central distribution)
- Hypertension or coronary heart disease
- Dyslipidaemia
- Physical inactivity

---

two people in the family with diabetes. Ethnic origin also dictates risk and in the United Kingdom the two main groups who have a higher risk of diabetes are Asian Indians, and Afro-Caribbeans, with both groups having fairly similar risks. In Newcastle, nearly 20% of Asian Indian adults had diabetes compared with 4% of Europeans.[4] A further 20–25% had impaired glucose tolerance, i.e. those at risk of developing type 2 diabetes mellitus. In Mauritius, in the Indian Ocean, many of the Chinese people had diabetes, whereas in Newcastle, the prevalence of diabetes in the Chinese was similar to Europeans. Therefore anyone from South Asia or anyone of Afro-Caribbean origin admitted to ICU, although they may not be admitted as a diabetic, may well turn out to have diabetes.

Another risk factor is obesity, particularly centrally distributed fat rather than that found peripherally. Abdominal obesity is common amongst males in particular. Risk factors for myocardial disease, such as hypertension and dyslipidaemia are also a significant risk factor for diabetic disease. Smoking, however, is not a particular risk factor for diabetes. The so-called deadly quintet for developing cardiovascular disease are diabetes or impaired glucose tolerance, dyslipidaemia, hypertension, obesity and smoking. In addition physical inactivity is a major modifiable risk factor.

Routine management

It is probably important to reiterate that in the management of patients with diabetes, education and self-monitoring are absolutely essential. If patients' selfcare is optimised, then we estimate that of patients with type 2 diabetes, up to 90% should be able to be managed with diet and exercise alone. It is therefore a sad reflection on us and others that in fact that figure is only about 20%. In the type 1 patient again education is very important since if a patient can learn a lot about their diabetes then they can have a much more flexible life.

Insulin

There are two categories of insulins (short-acting and intermediate-acting), and both types include porcine, human and modified human insulins. Genetically modified short-acting insulins act much more quickly since they are more rapidly absorbed and more closely mimic the normal meal-time profile. Long-acting modified human insulins to provide baseline levels are also appearing on the market.

Oral agents

The field of oral agents is changing rapidly and includes metformin and the sulphonureas, and newer agents such as repaglinide and thiazolodinediones (glitazones) and also glucosidase inhibitors. Some degree of hepatic toxicity has been reported for the glitazones but they are good at decreasing insulin resistance – a major factor in causing hyperglycaemia in type 2 diabetes.

Monitoring

In the last few months almost non-invasive glucose monitors have become available. A tiny needle under the skin, under a wristwatch-like machine, works through the microdialysis principle and provides a readout. There are several of these available and they could prove useful on the wards as well as for home monitoring.

Emergency management

Any diabetic patient who is not able to take food by mouth, the catabolic patient, those who are undergoing emergency surgery, and particularly people with myocardial infarction, ketoacidosis, hyperosmolar coma and people with low blood glucose, may arrive on the ICU (Box 4.2). It is safe to assume that type 1 diabetic patients have no insulin secretion, and that it must be replaced whatever else is happening to the patient. The mistake often made is that patients who are not eating do not need insulin, and that of course is untrue. In addition, patients who are very ill, particularly after surgery, will be insulin resistant as well. Type 2 patients already have sluggish insulin secretion and they can be very insulin resistant, worsened by any sort of stress. If a patient's blood glucose is 12 or even 15 mmol/L, the patient does not feel discomfort, but immune function and healing is impaired. The author's own plasma glucose target bracket in an acutely ill diabetic patient is a level of 6–10

Box 4.2 Diabetic patients: which patients are likely to be seen on ICU
- Nil-by-mouth
- Catabolic
- Surgical
- Myocardial infarction
- Diabetic ketoacidosis
- Hyperosmolar non-ketotic coma
- Hypoglycaemic coma

---

mmol/L. This is against a background of catabolic hormones, some of which will be inhibiting insulin secretion and most of which will be causing insulin resistance.

A basic management protocol, initially designed for diabetic patients undergoing surgery, can be used in a lot of different clinical situations for ill diabetic patients requiring intravenous insulin therapy (Table 4.5).[5] The basic therapy comprises 30–32 units insulin + 20 mmol potassium chloride in 1 litre 10% dextrose given 8 hourly. This can be modified according to patient need but in certain situations some patients will need more insulin. In patients with liver disease, particularly cirrhosis, there is insulin resistance and hence more insulin is needed. The same applies in major infection. A general guide to insulin requirements in the diabetic patients on ICU is given in Table 4.5. One situation where very large amounts of insulin are required is during cardiopulmonary bypass.

Table 4.5 Management of diabetes on ICU

- **Nil-by-mouth**
  Standard GKI
- **Catabolic**
  Parenteral nutrition + GKI
- **Surgical**
  Delay surgery until metabolically stable
  Frequent plasma glucose monitoring
  Omit glucose from GKI until plasma glucose <15 mmol/L
- **Myocardial infarction**
  Intravenous insulin first 24 hours
  Subcutaneous insulin 3–12 months
- **Diabetic ketoacidosis**
  Fluid
  Insulin
  Potassium
  Bicarbonate
  Other measures as needed

GKI = glucose–potassium–insulin: 1 litre 10% glucose, 32 units short-acting insulin, 20 mmol/L potassium chloride.

Table 4.6 Insulin requirements relative to glucose administration

Type of patient	Units insulin/g glucose
Uncomplicated	0.25–0.35
Liver disease	0.4–0.6
Obese	0.4–0.6
Sepsis	0.6–0.8
Steroid treatment	0.5–0.8
Cardiopulmonary bypass	>1.0

The insulin doses will require to be adjusted as plasma glucose changes. Glucose should be monitored about every 4 hours. An algorithm for adjusting insulin dose is given in Figure 4.1. It is important to remember that, unlike subcutaneous insulin, intravenous insulin has a half-life of only 4 minutes and if you stop the infusion even though the action goes on a little longer, you are stopping treating that patient. This is probably the commonest mistake and should be avoided. An often asked question is whether 5% or 10% glucose or saline–dextrose should be used. The author prefers 10% glucose to provide a few more calories. Certainly in patients with acute acidosis there is metabolic improvement in terms of ketones if 10% rather than 5% glucose is given. In catabolic patients receiving total parental nutrition glucose–potassium–insulin (GKI) can be administered in parallel, with intravenous nutrition going in the other arm (Table 4.5), but if the nutrition includes lipid, insulin resistance may be greater and the insulin in the GKI solution may need to be increased.

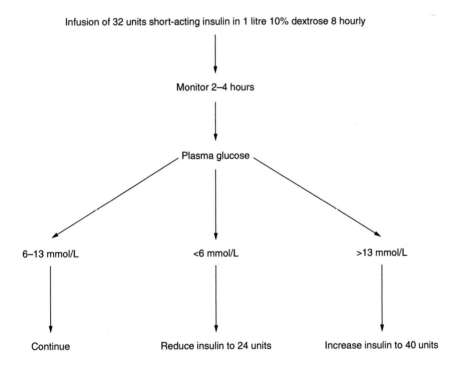

Infusion of 32 units short-acting insulin in 1 litre 10% dextrose 8 hourly

Monitor 2–4 hours

Plasma glucose

| 6–13 mmol/L | <6 mmol/L | >13 mmol/L |

| Continue | Reduce insulin to 24 units | Increase insulin to 40 units |

Note: Half-life of insulin is only 4 minutes: alter by 8–10 units/L per step and never stop insulin completely.

Figure 4.1   How to adjust insulin during intravenous glucose infusion.

In diabetic patients requiring emergency surgery, it is recommended that surgery is delayed if possible, particularly in those patients admitted with an acute abdomen who are also ketoacidotic, since many of the younger patients will resolve spontaneously as the metabolic abnormalities are corrected. In patients with myocardial infarction there has been some very interesting recent work suggesting that every diabetic patient with myocardial infarction should be treated with intravenous insulin. In the DIGAMI study,[6] intravenous insulin was administered to diabetic patients after myocardial infarction for the first 24 hours, followed by 3–5 months of subcutaneous insulin, whether it was required for glycaemic control or not (Table 4.5). Deaths were reduced by about 30%.

Patients with acute diabetic ketoacidosis are often seen on ICU, but one must remember that such patients may be unconscious for reasons other than diabetes. However diabetes may contribute in terms of ketoacidosis, hypoglycaemia or hyperosmolar coma. Such patients may develop acute respiratory distress syndrome or cerebral oedema, often due in part to the use by diabetologists, particularly paediatricians, of rapid hypotonic fluid replacement. Hyperosmolar non-ketotic coma is also not uncommon, particularly in type 2 diabetic patients, and older patients. Patients are admitted often with very high plasma glucose levels, and can be very dehydrated. About 10–15% of diabetic comas are hyperosmolar non-ketotic coma, precipitated by severe illness, dehydration, various drugs, total parenteral nutrition, haemodialysis or surgery. Hypoglycaemia occurs due to a mismatch between insulin dose, glucose or food intake and physical activity. Treatment is oral glucose, glucagon or intravenous glucose (20% glucose rather than 50% should be used).

Conclusion

New classification criteria for diabetes have lessened confusion in terminology and using the recommendations suggested in this article, the management of the diabetic patient admitted to the intensive care unit should be relatively straightforward, and errors in management should be prevented.

References

1 Alberti KG, Zimmet PZ. Definition, diagnosis and classification of diabetes and its complications. Part 1: diagnosis and classification of diabetes mellitus. Provisional report of a WHO consultation. *Diabetic Med* 1998;**15**:539–43.
2 Amos AF, McCarty DJ, Zimmet P. The rising global burden of diabetes and its complications: estimates and projections to the year 2010. *Diabetic Med* 1997;**14**:S1–S85.

3 DECODE Study Group on behalf of the European Diabetes Epidemiology Group. Consequences of the new diagnostic criteria for diabetes in older men and women. *Diabetes Care* 1999;**22:**1669–71.
4 Unwin N, Alberti KG, Bhopal R, *et al.* Comparison of the current WHO and new ADA criteria for the diagnosis of diabetes mellitus in three ethnic groups in the UK. *Diabetic Med* 1998;**15:**554–7.
5 Alberti KG. Diabetes and surgery. In: Pate D, Sherwin RS, eds. *Ellenberg and Rifkin's diabetes mellitus,* 5th edn, pp. 875–85. Stanford, Connecticut: Appleton and Lange, 1996.
6 Malmberg K, Ryden L, Efendic S, *et al.* Randomised controlled trial of insulin treatment in diabetic patients with acute myocardial infarction (DIGAMI Study): efforts on mortality at 1 year. *J Am Coll Cardiol* 1995;**26:**57–65.

5: Sex hormone-mediated modulation of the immune response after trauma, haemorrhage or sepsis

MARTIN G SCHWACHA, IRSHAD H CHAUDRY

Introduction

Despite significant improvements in preventative methods, and advances in patient care, trauma remains one of the leading causes of mortality during the first 30 years of life in the United States.[1,2] Trauma is a severe form of injury that includes bone fracture, penetrating soft-tissue injury (i.e. gunshot wounds), burn injury and prolonged surgical procedures. Many forms of traumatic injury can be associated with significant blood loss. In this regard, approximately 50% of the trauma related deaths are due to exsanguination or central nervous system complications during the initial 60-minute post-traumatic period. Moreover, during the following 2 hours, more than 30% of the patients die due to major internal organ damage.[3] The prognosis for the trauma patients who survive remains dire and approximately 50% of them die over the next few days to week(s) from secondary complications such as sepsis (an infection in the blood or other tissues with pathogenic microorganisms or toxins) and multiple-organ failure.[4-9] Sepsis is therefore a major non-neurological cause of death following trauma.[10] Much of the scientific and medical research has been, and remains, directed towards understanding the relationship between trauma and/or shock and the predisposition of these patients to septic/infectious complications and/or multiple-organ failure.[9,11-16]

The immune response to trauma, haemorrhage and sepsis

Both traumatic and haemorrhagic insults markedly alter immune status. These changes in immune status include suppressed polymorphonuclear

36

cell function, defective opsonisation, altered macrophage functions such as antigen presentation and cytokine production, suppression of T- and B-lymphocyte function (i.e. cytokine and antibody production, proliferation) and altered systemic pro- and anti-inflammatory mediator/cytokine patterns.[17-25] Immune dysfunction following trauma is believed to be a key factor in the development of sepsis and multiple-organ failure. Moreover, sepsis which is independent of an initiating insult such as trauma and/or haemorrhage also has profound deleterious effects on immunological functions.[26]

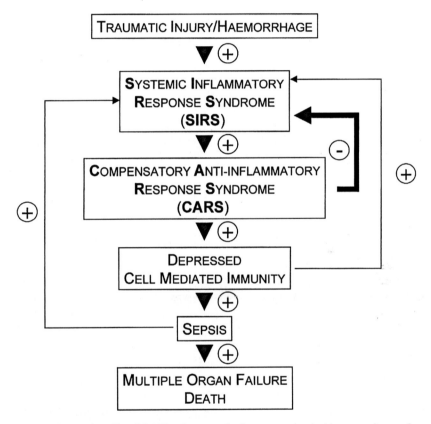

Figure 5.1 Schematic outline of the deleterious cascade of events associated with trauma, haemorrhage and sepsis. Traumatic injury or haemorrhage causes the activation of a pro-inflammatory cascade (SIRS) that includes TNF-α, IL-1β, and IL-6. SIRS is countered by an anti-inflammatory cascade (CARS) which includes IL-4, IL-10, TGF-β PGE$_2$. CARS acts to dampen the inflammatory response of SIRS. However, CARS is suppressive to many aspects of cell-mediated immunity which combats infection leading to immunosuppression and increased susceptibility to sepsis. The depression of cell-mediated immunity feeds back to activate SIRS which in turn further promotes CARS. The development of subsequent sepsis as a result of the immunosuppression mediated by CARS can act as a positive feedback on the cascade leading to multiple organ failure and death.

Traumatic injury and/or haemorrhage causes the activation of a network of pro-inflammatory responses that includes release of tumour necrosis factor-α (TNF-α), interleukin-1β (IL-1β) and IL-6, which are produced predominantly by macrophages. This is referred to as the systemic inflammatory response syndrome (SIRS).[4,27] This pro-inflammatory response is subsequently countered by an anti-inflammatory process called the compensatory anti-inflammatory response syndrome or "CARS". CARS is characterised by an early rise in systemic levels of the cyclooxygenase product prostaglandin (PG) E$_2$ which closely follows the initial increase in the pro-inflammatory cytokines IL-1β and IL-6 associated with SIRS. The rise in systemic PGE$_2$ is then subsequently followed by the cytokines transforming growth factor-α (TGF-α), IL-4 and IL-10. CARS acts to dampen the pro-inflammatory response of SIRS and represents the hosts attempt to bring itself back into an "immunological balance". When the immunological balance between SIRS and CARS is lost the effects can be deleterious to the host (Figure 5.1). With regard to immunologic responsiveness, CARS suppresses many aspects of cell-mediated immunity which combats infection. In addition, the depression of cell-mediated immunity feeds back to further promote SIRS. The CARS mediated-immune depression increases susceptibility to sepsis or other infections. If sepsis develops due to CARS-mediated immune depression, it can also stimulate SIRS which promotes CARS and further depresses cell-mediated immunity. Thus, the deleterious sequelae of SIRS, CARS and depressed cell-mediated immunity reinforce one another, ultimately leading to multiple-organ failure and death.

Gender and autoimmunity

Both clinical and experimental studies suggest that gender significantly influences immune function.[4,28-30] A remarkable preponderance of autoimmune diseases in females (i.e. systemic lupus erythematosus, Hashimoto's thyroiditis, rheumatoid arthritis), has been observed in both human and experimental studies.[30-32] Studies have also shown that by altering the sex hormone environment, the onset and course of autoimmune lupus in the F1 NZB/NZW mouse model can be modulated. Female F1 NZB/NZW mice normally develop the disease. However, administration of dihydrotestosterone prior to puberty prevents disease development, whereas castration of male mice has the opposite effect.[33,34] Further support for the concept that male and female sex hormones differently affect autoimmune disease processes comes from studies which demonstrate a correlation between lower androgen levels and increased oestrogen levels in women with systemic lupus erythematosus compared to age-matched healthy female controls.[35-37]

As early as 1898, Calzolari reported a connection between sex steroids and immune function.[38] More recent reports indicate a shorter skin allograft rejection time in females compared to males.[39] Furthermore, depletion of androgens in male animals by prior castration significantly shortens the time for skin rejection. In contrast to androgens, oestrogens can stimulate macrophage functions as evidenced by increased phagocytosis, cytokine production and antigen presentation.[40–43] Thus, a marked sexual dimorphism in immune function exists that appears to be related to gender-related differences in sex hormone levels.

The understanding of the mechanisms of action of sex hormones in both normal and pathological states has expanded dramatically due to the identification of specific receptors for these hormones and elucidation of the signal transduction cascade leading to cellular differentiation and division.[44] Steroid hormones (i.e. testosterone, oestrogen, progesterone) induce their biological effects by binding to a specific high-affinity receptor located in the target cell nucleus. Steroid hormones in combination with their specific receptors act as nuclear transcription factors which regulate gene expression. In the absence of ligand (i.e. sex steroid) the receptor is complexed with heat-shock proteins in an inactive state in the cell nucleus. Upon the binding of ligand to its specific receptor, the receptors become activated. The ligand–receptor complexes dimerize and release the heat-shock proteins. The ligand–receptor dimers are subsequently phosphorylated and bind to specific elements on DNA along with other regulatory proteins leading to gene activation.[44] In contrast to sex steroids, the female sex hormone prolactin does not act through nuclear receptors, but rather via more traditional membrane-bound receptors belonging to the cytokine receptor superfamily.[45] The binding of ligand to this type of receptor leads to the activation of the JAK-STAT family of tyrosine kinases followed by phosphorylation of specific cytosolic proteins and subsequent induction of gene transcriptional activity. While sex steroid receptors are located in the nucleus and prolactin receptors are membrane bound, their ultimate action following ligand binding is similar, namely gene activation. Thus, the action of all sex hormones on cellular functions is genomic, whether their action is direct (i.e. sex steroids) or indirect (i.e. prolactin).

Gender dimorphism in the immune response

Several epidemiological studies indicate the importance of gender as an additional risk factor for the development of sepsis and multiple-organ failure.[28,46] The majority of injured victims are young males[46–48] and they are more prone to septic complications after trauma than females.[4] Thus, gender differences exist in both the prevalence of trauma and the susceptibility to sepsis following such insults. McGowan *et al.* reported a

39

significantly higher incidence of bacteraemic infections in traumatised males than in female trauma patients.[28] Similarly, recent findings by Schröder *et al.* have shown a significantly higher survival rate in premenopausal women compared to men following the onset of sepsis.[49]

Experimental studies also indicate gender-related differences in the immune response following the induction of sepsis or sepsis-like states. Female mice in the proestrus state of their oestrus cycle, which is characterised by elevated oestrogen and prolactin levels, have been found to tolerate sepsis better than male mice, as demonstrated by markedly increased survival rates following a polymicrobial septic challenge.[50] This improved survival rate was associated with maintained splenocyte functions in females compared to depressed immune responses in male mice under those conditions. Moreover, female rates have been reported to be more resistant to lethal circulatory stress induced by trauma or intestinal ischaemia[51] and female mice in the proestrus state of the oestrus cycle have been found to exhibit enhanced splenic and peritoneal macrophage immune responses as opposed to depressed immune responses in males following trauma–haemorrhage.[52]

In an attempt to study the specific effects of testosterone and oestradiol under controlled experimental conditions, male mice were castrated 2 weeks prior to trauma–haemorrhage or sham operation and treated with placebo, 5α-dihydrotestosterone, 17β-oestradiol or a combination of both hormones.[53,54] The results of such studies indicated that: (i) splenic and peritoneal macrophage cytokine production was maintained in castrated male animals receiving placebo following trauma–haemorrhage; (ii) 5α-dihydrotestosterone treatment depressed splenic and peritoneal macrophages following trauma–haemorrhage to levels comparable to those encountered in non-castrated male mice; (iii) animals treated with 17β-oestradiol following castration had maintained or enhanced splenic and peritoneal macrophage function following trauma–haemorrhage and; (iv) the increased Kupffer cell cytokine production normally observed in males following trauma–haemorrhage was prevented by castration or 17β-oestradiol treatment, even in the presence of 5α-dihydrotestosterone. The generalised effect of testosterone and oestrogen treatment of castrated male mice on cytokine production by various macrophage populations following trauma–haemorrhage is summarized in Table 5.1. These finding suggest that the ratio of androgen to oestrogen may be an important factor in whether or not immunosuppression is observed following trauma–haemorrhage.

Thymic function (the thymus is the primary site of T-cell lymphopoiesis) is suppressed in male mice following trauma–haemorrhage due to decreased IL-3 secretion, which is important for T-lymphocyte maturation, and increased apoptosis (programmed cell death).[55] Gender dimorphism also exists in this primary lymphoid organ following haemorrhagic shock since

Table 5.1 Effect of 5α-dihydrotestosterone and 17β-oestradiol on macrophage cytokine release following trauma-haemorrhage in mice

Macrophage population	Cytokine	5α-Dihydrotestosterone	17β-Oestradiol
Splenic	IL-1β	–	No change
	IL-6	–	No change
	IL-10	+	–
Peritoneal	IL-1β	–	No change
	IL-6	–	No change
	IL-10	+	–
Hepatic	IL-1β	Not determined	Not determined
(Kupffer cells)	IL-6	+	No change
	IL-10	+	No change

Relative changes in the lipopolysaccharide stimulated release of pro- (IL-1β, IL-6) and anti- (IL-10) inflammatory cytokines by splenic peritoneal and hepatic (Kupffer cells) macrophages in 5α-dihydrotestosterone- and 17β-oestradiol-treated castrated male animals following trauma–haemorrhage as compared to sham mice treated with the same hormone concentrations. Data reproduced with permission from Angele *et al. Am J Physiol* 1999;277:C35–C42.[53]

(+) increased productive capacity; (–) decreased productive capacity.

proestus female did not display suppressed IL-3 secretion or increased apoptosis following trauma–haemorrhage.[56] Furthermore, *in vitro* treatment of thymocytes with 5α-dihydrotestosterone increased the apoptotic rate and decreased IL-3 release in a dose-dependent manner, suggesting that testosterone is responsible for the suppression in thymic function in males following trauma–haemorrhage. Thus, the suppression of T-lymphocyte function in males following haemorrhage may be in part due to changes in thymic function leading to alterations in T-lymphocyte selection and maturation.

With regard to T-lymphocyte phenotypes, proestrus female mice show enhanced release of IL-2 and interferon-γ (IFN-γ) by splenic T-lymphocytes compared to depressed release of these cytokines by similar cells from male mice following trauma–haemorrhage.[52] T-helper (Th) lymphocytes can be categorized according to their cytokine expression in two broad groups: Th-1 cytokines, which in general support cell mediated immunity and Th-2 cytokines, which support humoral immune responses. Figure 5.2 shows the relative roles and interrelationships of Th-1 and Th-2 cytokines on immune function. The differential induction of Th-lymphocytes expressing Th-1 (IL-2, IFN-γ) and/or Th-2 (IL-4, IL-10) is key to the regulation of both beneficial and pathological immune responses. In general, Th-1 cytokines are pro-inflammatory, induce cell-mediated immunity and macrophage activation. In contrast, Th-2 cytokines are anti-inflammatory, suppress macrophage function and induce humoral

41

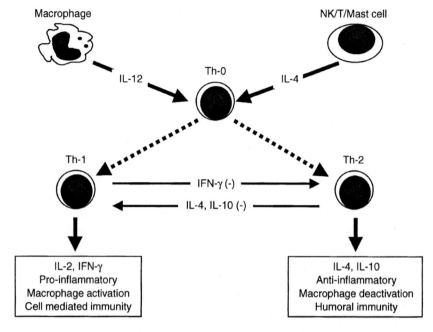

Figure 5.2 Interrelationship between Th-1 and Th-2 T-lymphocytes. Uncommitted T-lymphocytes (Th-0) differentiate into a Th-1 phenotype under the influence of macrophage derived IL-2 or a Th-2 phenotype under the influence of IL-4 derived from natural killer (NK), T- or mast cells. Th-1 cytokines (i.e. IL-2, IFN-γ) promote cell-mediated immune responses including macrophage activation. In general the response is pro-inflammatory. In contrast, Th-2 cytokines (i.e. IL-4, IL-10) promote humoral immunity and suppress macrophage function (deactivation). In general, the response is anti-inflammatory. Furthermore, both Th-1 and Th-2 cytokines have suppressive effects (–) on the development of their reciprocal T-lymphocyte phenotype.

immunity. Furthermore, Th-1 cytokines suppress Th-2 responses and Th-2 cytokines suppress Th-1 cytokines.

Ageing influences both T-lymphocyte phenotype and immune function. Studies have shown that the age-induced loss in protective immunity is primarily related to alterations in T-lymphocyte function.[57] In general, age-related changes in the production of T-lymphocyte cytokines are shifted to a Th-2 phenotype with ageing, as opposed to a predominance of the Th-1 phenotype in younger individuals.

Ageing also appears to reverse the gender dimorphism in infectious/septic complications following trauma. Schröder et al. reported that postmenopausal women had a higher mortality rate following sepsis than aged males.[49] In another retrospective study, McLauchlan et al. reviewed a group of patients with a mean age of 66 years who were admitted to the intensive care unit with abdominal sepsis.[58] The mortality rate of these patients was 63% and the factors associated with mortality included age and female gender. Moreover, Watanakunakorn's review of the medical records of patients who fulfilled the criteria for the diagnosis of *Staphylococcus aureus* endocarditis indicated that at age 60 or older, female gender was associated with higher mortality.[59] It is likely that the increased susceptibility to septic complications in aged females as compared to aged males is related to changes in circulating sex hormone levels.[60,61] The decrease in circulating oestrogens in the postmenopausal women appears to increase susceptibility to septic complications compared to premenopausal patients, whereas the decrease in circulating testosterone in aged males reduces susceptibility to such complications compared to younger patients.

Recent experimental findings indicate that the sexual dimorphism in T-lymphocyte responses following trauma–haemorrhage are reversed in aged animals.[62] Splenic T-lymphocyte responses (i.e. proliferation, IL-2 and IFN-γ release) were depressed in young male mice and enhanced in young females following trauma–haemorrhage. In contrast, in the aged male and female groups, these parameters of T-lymphocyte function were reversed following trauma–haemorrhage (i.e. increased proliferation and IL-2 release in aged males as compared to suppressed proliferation and IFN-γ release in aged females). Furthermore, the release of the Th-2 cytokine IL-10, inversely correlated with the age and gender related changes in splenic T-lymphocyte responses following trauma–haemorrhage. Similar to T-lymphocyte functions, gender dimorphism in macrophage function following trauma–haemorrhage is also influenced by aging.[63] Splenic and peritoneal macrophages from young female mice had enhanced IL-1β and suppressed IL-10 production following trauma–haemorrhage, whilst aged females had unchanged production IL-1β and IL-6 production and enhanced IL-10 release. In contrast, IL-1β and IL-6 production by macrophages from young males was suppressed and IL-10 production enhanced following trauma–haemorrhage whereas, cells from aged males produced elevated levels of IL-1β and IL-6 and suppressed levels of IL-10 following trauma–haemorrhage. These changes in immune function correlated with decreased testosterone in males and 17β-oestradiol in females with aging.

Immunomodulatory effects of sex hormones and related agents

Experimental studies have demonstrated that a number of sex hormones and related compounds such as receptor antagonists can modulate the immune response following traumatic injury, haemorrhagic shock and sepsis. These agents include oestradiol, dehydroepiandrosterone (DHEA), prolactin and prolactin-inducing agents such as the dopamine antagonist metoclopramide, and the testosterone receptor antagonist flutamide. The characteristics of these hormones/agents are outlined in Table 5.2.

43

Table 5.2 Sex hormones and related agents for restoration of immune function following trauma, haemorrhage or sepsis

Agent	Mode of action	Cellular effects	References
Oestradiol	Specific receptor activation	Nuclear binding and gene activation	41, 51, 68
Dehydroepiandosterone	Receptor activation	Oestrogenic agonist and glucocorticoid antagonist	78–82
Prolactin	Specific receptor activation	Protein kinase C activation and gene expression	86–90
Metoclopramide	Dopamine antagonist	Increase prolactin secretion	87, 94, 95
Flutamide	Androgen-receptor antagonist	Inhibition of androgen uptake and/or nuclear binding	96, 99

Although they have not yet been approved for clinical application in trauma patients, the experimental findings show promise in yielding safe, relatively inexpensive and useful approaches to alleviate the immune dysfunction associated with traumatic injury.

Oestrogen

In contrast to androgens, female sex steroids have immunostimulatory effects on cell-mediated immunity.[64] Oestrogens can stimulate macrophage functions, such as Fc receptor-mediated phagocytosis and IL-1β production.[41,65] Peripheral T-lymphocyte activity has also been reported to be modulated by oestrogen treatment either by enhancing the helper/inducer activity or suppressing suppressor/cytotoxic activity.[32,66] The alterations in immune function following oestrogen administration induce increased resistance to infection, lethal trauma or intestinal ischemia.[51,64,67] Knöferl et al. have shown that administration of a single dose of 17β-oestradiol to male mice following trauma–haemorrhage normalized plasma IL-6 levels.[68] Additionally, splenic T-lymphocyte IL-2 and IL-3 release and splenic macrophage IL-1 and IL-6 was not suppressed in 17β-oestradiol treated animals under such conditions. In contrast, the production of the immunosuppressive Th-2 cytokine IL-10 by splenic T-lymphocytes and macrophages following trauma–haemorrhage was reduced in the oestradiol-treated group. Further support for the role of oestradiol as an immunomodulatory agent following trauma comes from experimental studies in ovariectomized female mice. Such mice were immunosuppressed following trauma–haemorrhage, whereas intact animals in the proestrus state of the oestrus cycle had maintained immune function under such

44

conditions.[69] Ovariectomized female mice were also more susceptible to the deleterious consequences of polymicrobial sepsis following trauma–haemorrhage than their intact counterparts.

Dehydroepiandrosterone (DHEA)

DHEA is the most abundant steroid produced by the adrenals.[70] Whether or not it is a member of a distinct group of steroid hormones that possess unique physiological actions is unclear. DHEA is often called an "adrenal androgen" because it can be converted to testosterone in the periphery. Nonetheless, it is an intermediate in the pathway for the synthesis of both testosterone and oestrogen (Figure 5.3). In this regard, it

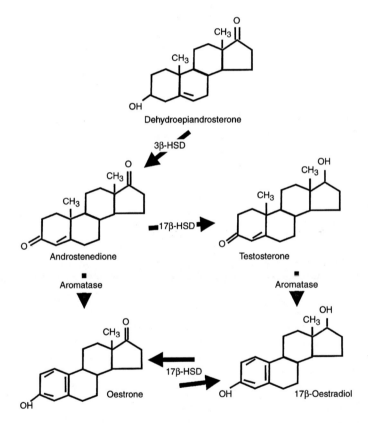

Figure 5.3 Dehydroepiandosterone (DHEA) as an intermediate in the biosynthesis of both sex steroid biosynthesis. DHEA is converted to androstenedione via the action of the enzyme 3β-hydroxysteroid dehydrogenase (3β-HSD). The intermediate is under the influence of two enzymes: (i) aromatase and (ii) 17β-hydroxysteroid dehydrogenase (17β-HSD). Aromatase acts to convert androstenedione to oestrone which can be subsequently converted to 17β-oestradiol by the action of 17β-HSD. 17β-HSD action on androstenedione converts it to testosterone. Testosterone can also be converted to 17β-oestradiol by the action of aromatase.

45

has been suggested that in the male hormonal environment, DHEA has predominantly oestrogenic affects.[71] However, evidence also supports the concept that the immunomodulatory actions of DHEA are direct, since the existence of specific DHEA receptors in lymphoid tissues has been reported.[72,73] DHEA has immunopotentiating action in both experimental animals and humans. It has been shown to improve the immune system of older animals and those treated with high doses of androgen.[74,75] DHEA has also been reported to decrease the mortality rate in animals infected with various viruses and bacteria.[76] Th-1 T-lymphocyte responses (Figure 5.2) have been reported to be stimulated by DHEA, thus potentially enhancing cell-mediated immune responses.[77]

Administration of DHEA to male mice following trauma–haemorrhage normalised various aspects of cell-mediated immunity as evidenced by maintained splenic and peritoneal macrophage and splenic T-lymphocyte cytokine production.[70,78] DHEA treatment of male mice following trauma–haemorrhage also significantly improved the survival rate of animals subjected to subsequent sepsis.[79] Araneo et al. have demonstrated that DHEA treatment of mice prevented the suppression of splenic immune functions following thermal injury.[80] Furthermore, in vitro treatment of splenocytes isolated from thermally injured mice with DHEA restored T-lymphocyte cytokine production to normal levels. In this study, in vivo treatment of injured mice with DHEA not only prevented the suppression in T-lymphocyte cytokine production, but also prevented the suppression in contact hypersensitivity and increased resistance to Listeria monocytogenes infection postburn.

The precise mechanisms underlying the immunostimulatory effects of DHEA are unresolved. Whilst DHEA-specific receptors have been identified on lymphocytes suggesting a direct action on immune cells,[72,73] other studies support the notion that the immunostimulatory action of DHEA is mediated via the oestrogen receptor. In this respect, Catania et al. reported that tamoxifen, an oestrogen-receptor antagonist, blocked the immunostimulatory effects of DHEA on mouse splenic T-lymphocytes in vitro.[78] In addition, DHEA may also modulate immune responses indirectly by antagonising some of the immunosuppressive effects of glucocorticoids.[81,82] The observation that DHEA administration to mice following trauma–haemorrhage normalised the elevated plasma glucocorticoid levels further supports the concept that the immunostimulatory action of DHEA is through suppression of glucocorticoid production.[78] Thus, DHEA might improve or restore cell-mediated immune responses following trauma, haemorrhage or sepsis indirectly by antagonising glucocorticoid-mediated immune depression. Whether the immunostimulatory action of DHEA is direct via DHEA-specific receptors, indirect via oestrogen receptors, or acts via suppression of glucocorticoid levels or indeed involves all these actions, remains to be resolved. Nonetheless, experimental studies clearly support DHEA as a potent immunomodulatory agent that may be useful in restoring immune function following trauma, irrespective of the mode of action.

Prolactin and the dopamine antagonist metoclopramide

The physiological release of prolactin from the pituitary fluctuates in a pulsatile circadian fashion, as do glucocorticoids, and is further modulated by behavioural and environmental stimuli, the reproductive cycle, steroid hormones, neurotransmitters, immunoregulatory cytokines and various drugs. Recent studies indicate that the immune system is an important target site for prolactin. Increasing evidence supports the notion that immune cells have specific receptors for prolactin, indicating a direct action of this sex hormone on such cells.[40] Prolactin may be a key hormone contributing to the dichotomy seen in the immune response between females and males.[83,84] In this regard, increased plasma concentrations of prolactin in females are associated with increased T-lymphocyte activity.[85] The increased T-helper and T-cytotoxic lymphocyte activity results in an increased cell-mediated immune response, accompanied by an increase in humoral immunity. Furthermore, the immune depression associated with chronic morphine treatment can be reversed by prolactin treatment, whereas pharmacological suppression of prolactin secretion in rodents has been shown to derange normal lymphocyte function and depress lymphocyte dependent host defences.[86] Thus considerable evidence exists implicating prolactin as an immunomodulatory hormone.

Treatment of septic male mice with prolactin after the onset of sepsis has been shown to result in significantly increased innate and inducible IL-1β, IL-6 and TNF-α gene expression in splenic and peritoneal macrophages as well as Kupffer cells.[87] Furthermore, the inducible gene expression for IL-1β and IL-6 by splenic and peritoneal macrophages from male mice following haemorrhage was also increased; however, the productive capacity for these cytokines was suppressed.[88] Prolactin administration following haemorrhage, corrected splenic and peritoneal macrophage IL-1β and IL-6 gene expression as well as the elevated Kupffer cell gene expression for IL-1β, IL-6, TNF-α and TGF-1β.[89] The suppression in T-lymphocyte responses following severe haemorrhage were also restored by prolactin treatment.[90] Administration of this immunomodulatory hormone following haemorrhage also decreased mortality from subsequent polymicrobial sepsis.[88]

Metoclopramide is frequently used in the clinical arena to alleviate nausea and vomiting that occurs in patients after surgery as well as in cancer patients and no major adverse effects have been reported. Metoclopramide administration has also been shown to increase prolactin secretion.[91] The increase in prolactin secretion is apparently the result of central antagonism of dopamine in the hypothalamus by metoclopramide. The relationship between the hypothalamic–pituitary–adrenal axis and immune function is shown in Figure 5.4. Further support for the interaction of the hypothalamic–pituitary–adrenal axis comes from studies reporting that opioids stimulate prolactin release and that the β-endorphin-mediated suppression of cortisol secretion in stressed animals is mediated by prolactin.[92,93]

Based on the findings that administration of prolactin after haemorrhagic shock restored the depressed immune responses, metoclopramide was administered following trauma–haemorrhage.[87,94] A single dose of metoclopramide following resuscitation normalised splenocyte IL-2 and

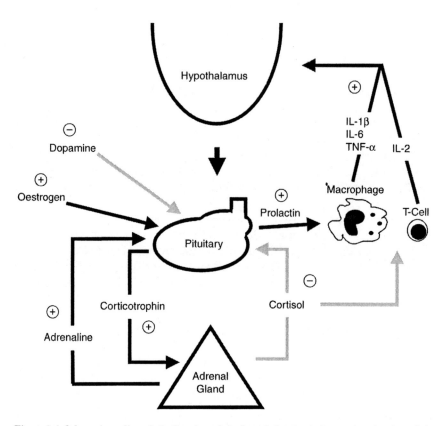

Figure 5.4 Schematic outline of the function of the hypothalamic–pituitary–adrenal axis and its relationship to immune function. The system includes negative-feedback loops: (i) cortisol feedback to control the output of corticotrophin by the pituitary and (ii) cytokines produced by immune cells act on the hypothalamus to upregulate cortisol release. Stimulation of the pituitary either by oestrogens or via the hypothalamus stimulates prolactin secretion which in turn stimulates immune cell function. Prolactin release is regulated by cortisol as described above as well as dopamine.

IL-3 release and treated animals exhibited normal peritoneal macrophage cytokine release patterns.[94] Similarly, administration of metoclopramide normalised the cytokine gene expression by splenic and peritoneal macrophages following the induction of polymicrobial sepsis.[87]

The mechanism by which metoclopramide normalises immune responses following haemorrhage appears to be related to its ability to increase plasma prolactin levels by blocking antagonistic effect of dopamine on the anterior pituitary. Recent studies support this notion, since prolactin, but not metoclopramide, added to *in vitro* cultures of splenocytes and macrophages from haemorrhaged mice corrected various immune parameters.[95] An additional mode of action of metoclopramide, however, has been reported by Zellweger *et al.* since metoclopramide administration following haemorrhage also normalised the elevated plasma corticosterone levels.[94] Thus, beneficial immunological effects of metoclopramide may relate to increasing prolactin secretion as well as suppression of glucocorticoid release.

The testosterone receptor antagonist flutamide

Studies have shown that the male sex hormone testosterone can suppress immune function in normal animals.[42] Furthermore, depletion of male sex steroids by prior castration can prevent the immunosuppression following haemorrhagic shock in young male mice,[53,96] as well as normalise the increased pro-inflammatory cytokine release by Kupffer cells which is normally observed under such conditions.[97] These findings implicate a role for testosterone in the regulation of immune function and suggest that testosterone is critical to the immune dysfunction observed in males following trauma.

Castration of male trauma victims to deplete plasma testosterone levels is obviously neither practical nor advocated. However, experimental studies indicate that temporary pharmacological castration using the androgen-receptor antagonist flutamide has beneficial affects on immune function in males following haemorrhagic shock. Flutamide is used clinically for the treatment of androgen-sensitive prostatic carcinoma. It is a non-steroidal agent which has potent anti-androgenic activity by inhibiting androgen uptake or nuclear binding of the activated androgen receptor to nuclear response elements in the nucleus. Flutamide has been shown to mimic the immune-enhancing effects of castration on B-lymphocyte function in male mice as evidenced by acceleration of autoimmune disease processes.[98] Flutamide treatment after trauma–haemorrhage has been shown to normalise the depressed macrophage function observed in male mice under such conditions.[96] Additionally administration of flutamide for three consecutive days following haemorrhage and resuscitation restored immune function even after the induction of subsequent sepsis. Such treatment also decreased the susceptibility of haemorrhaged animals to mortality associated with a subsequent septic challenge.[99] Therefore, since flutamide is used clinically for longer periods of time in the treatment of prostate cancer without major adverse effects, the short-term treatment of male trauma patients with flutamide might offer a safe, novel and useful approach for preventing immune dysfunction under those conditions.

Another common anti-androgenic compound is bucalutamide. It is non-steroidal and related to flutamide in its mechanism of action. Interestingly it is approximately 50 times more potent than flutamide in dogs, causing atrophy of the prostate, and has a 4-fold higher affinity for the androgen receptor. Unlike flutamide, which can elevate circulating testosterone levels, bucalutamide has little effect on serum testosterone.[100] Nonetheless, although the use of bucalutamide is promising in models of male trauma, efficacy studies have yet to be conducted.

Summary and conclusions

Despite the fact that clinical studies have shown that gender affects morbidity and mortality after trauma, haemorrhage and sepsis, alterations in immune status under such conditions have been studied primarily in animals. Only recently have clinical studies begun to investigate the effect of gender, age, and sex hormones on immune responses. In general, findings suggest that testosterone is immunosuppressive following traumatic injury, whereas the female sex hormones oestradiol and prolactin are protective under such conditions. The specific underlying mechanism(s) for the immunomodulatory properties of sex hormones on cell-mediated immune responses remains to be fully elucidated. Experimental evidence supports both direct and indirect effects in modulating the immune response. In this respect, sex hormone receptors have been identified on various immune cells, suggesting receptor-mediated processes. Other studies suggest the release of secondary mediators which alter immune responses. In view of those findings, clinically relevant therapeutic strategies have been developed using oestrogens, DHEA, prolactin and dopamine antagonists which enhance prolactin secretion, and testosterone receptor antagonists (Table 5.2). These agents may represent safe, useful, novel and relatively inexpensive therapeutic approaches for the treatment of immune dysfunction in trauma victims.

Acknowledgments

This work was supported by United States Public Health Service grant R01 GM 37127.

References

1   Shires GT. Principles and management of hemorrhagic shock. In: Shires GT, ed. *Principles of trauma care.* New York: McGraw-Hill, 1985.
2   Trunkey DD. Trauma. *Sci Amer* 1983;**249:**28–35.
3   Lewis FR, Krupski WC, Trunkey DD. Management of the injured patient. In: Way LW, ed. *Current surgical diagnosis and treatment.* San Mateo, CA: Appleton and Lange, 1988.
4   Bone RC. Toward an epidemiology and natural history of SIRS (systemic inflammatory response syndrome). *JAMA* 1992;**268:**3452–5.
5   Baue AE, Durham R, Faist E. Systemic inflammatory response syndrome (SIRS), multiple organ dysfunction syndrome (MODS), multiple organ failure (MOF): are we winning the battle? *Shock* 1998;**10:**79–89.
6   Cerra FB. Multiple organ failure syndrome. In: Bihari DJ, Cerra FB, ed. *Multiple organ failure.* Fullerton, CA: Society of Critical Care Medicine, 1989.
7   Deitch EA. *Multiple organ failure: pathophysiology and basic concepts of therapy.* New York: Thieme Medical Publishers, 1990.
8   Goris RJA. Sepsis and multiple organ failure: The result of whole body inflammation. In: Faist E, Meakins J, Schildberg FW, eds. *Host defence dysfunction in trauma, shock and sepsis.* Berlin and Heidelberg: Springer-Verlag, 1993.
9   Fry DE, Pearlstein L, Fulton RL, Polk HC, Jr. Multiple system organ failure. The role of uncontrolled infection. *Arch Surg* 1980;**115:**136–40.
10 Baker CC, Oppenheimer L, Lewis FR, Trunkey DD. The epidemiology of trauma death. *Am J Surg* 1980;**140:**144–50.
11 Alexander JW, Steinnett JD, Ogle CK, *et al.* A comparison of immunologic profiles and their influence on bacteremia in surgical patients with a high risk of infections. *Surgery* 1979;**86:**94–101.
12 Bjornson AB, Altemeir WA, Bjornson HS, *et al.* Host defence against opportunistic micro-organisms following trauma: studies to determine the association between changes in humoral components of host defense and septicemia in burned patients. *Ann Surg* 1978;**188:**93–101.
13 Border JR, Bone LB. Multiple trauma: major extremity wounds; their immediate management and its consequences. *Adv Surg* 1987;**21:**263–91.
14 Christou NV, MacLean L, Meakins JL. Host defense in blunt trauma: interrelationships of kinetics of anergy and depressed neutrophil function: nutritional status and sepsis. *J Trauma* 1980;**20:**833–41.
15 Baker CC, Degutis LC, DeSantis JG, Baue AE. The impact of a trauma service in a University Hospital. *Am J Surg* 1985;**149:**453–8.
16 Polk HC. Consensus summary on infections. *J Trauma* 1979;**19:**894–6.
17 Schwacha MG, Knöferl MW, Samy TSA, *et al.* The immunologic consequences of hemorrhagic shock. *Crit Care Shock* 1999;**2:**42–64.
18 Sayeed MM. Alterations in cell signalling and related effector functions in T lymphocytes in burn/trauma/sepsis injuries. *Shock* 1996;**5:**157–66.
19 Ayala A, Ertel W, Chaudry IH. Trauma-induced suppression of antigen presentation and expression of major histocompatibility class II antigen complex in leukocytes. *Shock* 1996;**5:**79–90.
20 Zellweger R, Ayala A, DeMaso CM, Chaudry IH. Trauma-hemorrhage causes prolonged depression in cellular immunity. *Shock* 1995;**4:**149–53.
21 Simms HH, D'Amico R. Polymorphonuclear leukocyte dysregulation during the systemic inflammatory response syndrome. *Blood* 1994;**83:**1398–407.

22 Schwacha MG, Somers SD. Thermal injury-induced immunosuppression in mice: the role of macrophage-derived reactive nitrogen intermediates. *J Leukoc Biol* 1998;**63**:51–8.

23 Schwacha MG, Ayala A, Cioffi WG, et al. Role of protein kinase C in cyclic AMP-mediated suppression of T-lymphocyte activation following burn injury. *Biochim Biophys Acta* 1999;**1455**:45–53.

24 Moss NM, Gough DB, Jordan AL, et al. Temporal correlation of impaired immune response after thermal injury with susceptibility to infection in a murine model. *Surgery* 1988;**104**:882–7.

25 O'Riordain MGT, Collins KH, Pilz M, et al. Modulation of macrophage hyperactivity improves survival in a burn–sepsis model. *Arch Surg* 1992;**127**:152–8.

26 Ayala A, Chaudry IH. Immune dysfunction in murine polymicrobial sepsis: mediators, macrophages, lymphocytes and apoptosis. *Shock* 1996;**6**:S27–S38.

27 Schlag G, Redl H, Bahrami S. SIRS (systemic inflammatory response syndrome) following trauma and during sepsis. *Anästhesiol Intensivmed Nötfallmed Schmerzther* 1994;**29**:37–41.

28 McGowan JE, Barnes MW, Finland N. Bacteremia at Boston City Hospital: occurrence and mortality during 12 selected years (1935–1972) with special reference to hospital-acquired cases. *J Infect Dis* 1975;**132**:316–35.

29 Terres G, Morrison SL, Habicht GS. A quantitative difference in the immune response between male and female mice. *Proc Soc Exp Biol Med* 1968;**127**:664–7.

30 Olsen NJ, Kovacs WJ. Gonadal steroids and immunity. *Endocrin Rev* 1996;**17**:369–84.

31 Viselli SM, Stanziale S, Shults K, et al. Castration alters peripheral immune function in normal male mice. *Immunology* 1995;**84**:337–42.

32 Roubinian JR, Talal N, Greenspan JS, et al. Effect of castration and sex hormone treatment on survival, anti-nucleic acid antibodies, and glomerulonephritis in NZB/NZW F1 mice. *J Exp Med* 1978;**147**:1568–83.

33 Roubinian JR, Talal N, Greenspan JS, et al. Delayed androgen treatment prolongs survival in murine lupus. *J Clin Invest* 1979;**63**:902–11.

34 Roubinian JR, Talal N, Siiteri PK, Sadakin JA. Sex hormone modulation for autoimmunity in NZB/NZW mice. *Arthritis Rheum* 1979;**22**:1162–9.

35 Junger WG, Nahoul K, Pelissier C, et al. Low plasma androgens in women with active or quiescent systemic lupus erythematosus. *Arthritis Rheum* 1982;**25**:454–7.

36 Lahita RG, Bradlow HL, Fishman J, Kunkel HG. Abnormal estrogen and androgen metabolism in humans with systemic lupus erythematosus. *Am J Kidney Dis* 1982;**2**:206–11.

37 Lahita RG, Bradlow HL, Ginzler E, et al. Low plasma androgens in women with systemic lupus erythematosus. *Arthritis Rheum* 1987;**30**:241–8.

38 Calzolari A. Recherches expérimentales sur un rapport probable entre la function du thymus et celle des testicules. *Arch Ital Biol* 1898;**30**:71–7.

39 Graff RJ, Lappe MA, Snell GD. The influence of gonads and adrenal glands on the immune response to skin grafts. *Transplantation* 1969;**7**:105–11.

40 Gala RR. Prolactin and growth hormone in the regulation of the immune system. *Proc Soc Exp Biol Med* 1991;**198**:513–27.

41 Hu SK, Mitcho ML, Rath NC. Effect of estradiol on interleukin-1 synthesis by macrophages. *Int J Immunopharm* 1988;**10**:247–52.

42 Weinstein Y, Ran S, Segal S. Sex-associated differences in the regulation of immune responses controlled by the MHC of the mouse. *J Immunol* 1984;**132**:656–61.

43 Wira CR, Rossoll RM. Antigen-presenting cells in the female reproductive tract: influence of sex hormones on antigen presentation in the vagina. *Immunology* 1995;**84**:505–8.

44 Beato M, Chavez S, Truss M. Transcriptional regulation by steroid hormones. *Steroids* 1996;**61**:240–51.

45 Wells JA, De Vos AM. Hematopoietic receptor complexes. *Ann Rev Biochem* 1996;**65**:609–34.

46 Feero S, Hedges JR, Simmons E, Irwin L. Intracity regional demographics of major trauma. *Ann Emerg Med* 1995;**25**:788–93.

47 Kong LB, Lekawa M, Navarro RA, *et al.* Pedestrian–motor vehicle trauma: an analysis of injury profiles by age. *J Am Coll Surg* 1996;**182**:17–23.

48 Williams JM, Furbee PM, Prescott JE, Paulson DJ. The emergency department log as a simple injury-surveillance tool. *Ann Emerg Med* 1995;**25**:686–91.

49 Schröder J, Kahlke V, Staubach KH, *et al.* Gender differences in human sepsis. *Arch Surg* 1998;**133**:1200–5.

50 Zellweger R, Ayala A, Stein S, *et al.* Females in proestus state tolerate sepsis better than males. *Crit Care Med* 1997;**25**:106–10.

51 Altura BM. Sex and estrogens in protection against circulatory stress reactions. *Am J Physiol* 1976;**231**:842–7.

52 Wichmann MW, Zellweger R, DeMaso CM, *et al.* Enhanced immune responses in females as opposed to decreased responses in males following hemorrhagic shock. *Cytokine* 1996;**8**:853–63.

53 Angele MK, Knöferl M, Schwacha MG, *et al.* Testosterone and estrogen regulate pro- and antiinflammatory cytokine release by macrophages following trauma-hemorrhage. *Am J Physiol* 1999;**277**:C35–C42.

54 Angele MK, Ayala A, Monfils BA, *et al.* Testosterone and/or low estradiol: normally required but harmful immunologically for males after trauma-hemorrhage. *J Trauma* 1998;**44**:78–85.

55 Xu YX, Wichmann MW, Ayala A, *et al.* Trauma-hemorrhage induces increased thymic apoptosis while decreasing IL-3 release and increasing GM-CSF. *J Surg Res* 1997;**68**:24–30.

56 Angele MK, Xin Xu Y, Ayala A, *et al.* Gender differences in immune responses: Increased thymocyte apoptosis occurs only in males but not in females after trauma-hemorrhage. *Shock* 1999;**12**:316–22.

57 Miller RA. The aging immune system: primer and prospectus. *Science* 1996;**273**:70–4.

58 McLauchlan GJ, Anderson ID, Grant IS, Fearon KC. Outcome of patients with abdominal sepsis treated in an intensive care unit. *Br J Surg* 1995;**82**:524–9.

59 Watanakunakorn C. *Staphylococcus aureus* endocarditis at a community teaching hospital, 1980 to 1991. An analysis of 106 cases. *Arch Int Med* 1994;**154**:2330–5.

60 Wich BK, Carnes M. Menopause and the aging female reproductive system. *Endo Metab Clin N Am* 1995;**24**:273–95.

61 Tsitouras P, Bulat T. The aging male reproductive system. *Endo Metab Clin N Am* 1995;**24**:297–315.

62 Kahlke V, Angele MK, Schwacha MG, *et al.* Reversal of sexual dimorphism in

splenic T-lymphocyte responses following trauma-hemorrhage with aging. *Am J Physiol* (in press).

63 Kahlke V, Angele MK, Ayala A, *et al.* Immune dysfunction following trauma-hemorrhage: influence of gender and age. *Cytokine* 2000;**12**:69–77.

64 Yamamoto Y, Saito H, Setogawa T, Tomioka H. Sex differences in host resistance to *Mycobacterium marinum* infection in mice. *Infect Immun* 1991;**59**:4089–96.

65 Friedman D, Netti F, Schreiber AD. Effect of estradiol and steroid analogues on the clearance of immunoglobulin G-coated erythrocytes. *J Clin Invest* 1985;**75**:162–7.

66 Carlsten H, Tarkowski A, Holmdahl R, Nilsson LA. Oestrogen is a potent disease accelerator in SLE-prone MRL 1pr/1pr mice. *Clin Exp Immunol* 1990;**80**:467–73.

67 Nicol T, Bilbey DLJ, Charles LM, *et al.* Oestrogen: the natural stimulant of body defense. *J Endocrinol* 1964;**30**:277–91.

68 Knöferl MW, Diodato MD, Angele MK, *et al.* Do female sex steroids adversely or beneficially affect the depressed immune responses in males following trauma-hemorrhage? *Arch Surg* 2000;**135(4)**:425–33.

69 Knöferl MW, Angele MK, Diodato MD, *et al.* Surgical ovariectomy produces immunodepression following trauma–hemorrhage and increases mortality from susbequent sepsis. *Surg Forum* 1999;**50**:235–7.

70 Svec F, Porter JR. The actions of exogenous dehydroepiandrosterone in experimental animals and humans. *Proc Soc Exp Biol Med* 1998;**218**:174–91.

71 Ebeling P, Koivisto VA. Physiological importance of dehydroepiandrosterone. *Lancet* 1994;**343**:1479–81.

72 Okabe T, Haji M, Takayanagi R, *et al.* Upregulation of high-affinity dehydroepiandosterone binding activity by dehydroepiandosterone in activated human T lymphocytes. *J Clin Endocrinol Metab* 1995;**80**:2993–6.

73 Meikle AW, Dorchuck RW, Araneo BA, *et al.* The presence of a dehydreoepiandrosterone-specific receptor binding complex in murine T cells. *J Steroid Biochem Molec Biol* 1992;**42**:293–304.

74 Garg M, Bondada S. Reversal of age-associated decline in immune response to Pnu-immune vaccine by supplementation with the steroid hormone dehydroepiandrosterone. *Infect Immun* 1993;**61**:2238–41.

75 Kim HR, Ryu SY, Kim HS, *et al.* Administration of dehydroepiandrosterone reverses the immune suppression induced by high dose antigen. *Immunol Invest* 1995;**24**:583–93.

76 Loria RMRW, Padgett DA. Immune response facilitation and resistance to virus and bacterial infections with dehydroepiandrosterone (DHEA). In: Kalimi M, Regalson W, eds. *The biological role of dehydroepiandrosterone (DHEA)*. New York: Walter De Gruyter, 2000.

77 Daynes RA, Dudley DJ, Araneo BA. Regulation of murine lymphokine production *in vivo*. II. Dehydroepiandrosterone is a natural enhancer of interleukin 2 synthesis by helper T cells. *Eur J Immunol* 1990;**20**:793–802.

78 Catania RA, Angele MK, Ayala A, *et al.* Dehydroepiandrosterone restores immune function following trauma–haemorrhage by a direct effect on T lymphocytes. *Cytokine* 1999;**11**:443–50.

79 Angele MK, Catania RA, Ayala A, *et al.* Dehydroepiandrosterone: an inexpensive steroid hormone that decreases the mortality due to sepsis following trauma-induced hemorrhage. *Arch Surg* 1998;**133**:1281–8.

80 Araneo BA, Shelby J, Li GZ, *et al.* Administration of dehydroepiandrosterone

to burned mice preserves normal immunologic competence. *Arch Surg* 1993;**128**:318–25.

81 Araneo BA, Shelby J, Li G, *et al*. Dehydroepiandrosterone antagonizes the suppressive effects of dexamethasone on lymphocyte proliferation. *Arch Surg* 1993;**128**:318–25.

82 Blauer KL, Poth M, Rogers WM, Bernton EW. Dehydroepiandrosterone antagonizes the suppressive effects of dexamethasone on lymphocyte proliferation. *Endocrinology* 1997;**129**:3174–9.

83 Shen GK, Montgomery DW, Ulrich ED, *et al*. Up-regulation of prolactin gene expression and feedback modulation of lymphocyte proliferation during acute allograft rejection. *Surgery* 1992;**112**:387–94.

84 Athreya BH, Pletcher J, Zulian F, *et al*. Subset-specific effects of sex hormones and pituitary gonadotropins on human lymphocyte proliferation *in vitro*. *Clin Immunol Immunopathol* 1993;**66**:201–11.

85 Grossman C. Possible underlying mechanisms of sexual dimorphism in the immune response. Fact and hypothesis. *J Steroid Biochem* 1989;**34**:241–51.

86 Bernton EW. Prolactin and immune host defences. *Prog Neuroendocrine Immunol* 1989;**2**:21–9.

87 Zhu X-H, Zellweger R, Wichmann MW, *et al*. Effects of prolactin and metoclopramide on macrophage cytokine gene expression in late sepsis. *Cytokine* 1997;**9**:437–46.

88 Zellweger R, Zhu X-H, Wichmann MW, *et al*. Prolactin administration following hemorrhagic shock improves macrophage cytokine release capacity and decreases mortality from subsequent sepsis. *J Immunol* 1996;**157**:5748–54.

89 Zhu X-H, Zellweger R, Ayala A, Chaudry IH. Prolactin inhibits the increased cytokine gene expression in Kupffer cells following haemorrhage. *Cytokine* 1996;**8**:134–40.

90 Zellweger R, Wichmann MW, Ayala A, *et al*. Prolactin: a novel and safe immunomodulating hormone for the treatment of immunodepression following severe hemorrhage. *J Surg Res* 1996;**63**:53–8.

91 Ehrenkranz RA, Ackerman BA. Metoclopramide effect on faltering milk production by mothers of premature infants. *Pediatrics* 1986;**78**:614–20.

92 Parrott RF, Goode JA. Central effects of naloxone and selected opioid agonists on cortisol and prolactin secretion in non-stressed sheep. *Gen Pharmacol* 1993;**24**:101–3.

93 Domanski E, Romanowicz K, Kerdelhué B. Enhancing effect of intracerebrally inflused β-endorphin antiserum on the secretion of cortisol in foot-shocked sheep. *Neuroendocrinology* 1993;**57**:127–31.

94 Zellweger R, Wichmann MW, Ayala A, Chaudry IH. Metoclopramide: A novel and safe immunomodulating agent for restoring the depressed macrophage function following trauma-hemorrhage. *J Trauma* 1998;**44**:70–7.

95 Knöferl MW, Angele MK, Ayala A, *et al*. Insights into the mechanism by which metoclopramide improves immune functions following trauma-hemorrhage. *Am J Physiol* (in press).

96 Wichmann MW, Angele MK, Ayala A, *et al*. Flutamide: A novel agent for restoring the depressed cell-mediated immunity following soft-tissue trauma and hemorrhagic shock. *Shock* 1997;**8**:1–7.

97 Ayala A, Perrin MM, Ertel W, Chaudry IH. Differential effects of haemorrhage on Kupffer cells: decreased antigen presentation despite increased inflammatory cytokine (IL-1, IL-6 and TNF) release. *Cytokine* 1992;**4**:66–75.

98 Walker SE, Besch-Williford CL, Keisler DH. Accelerated deaths from systemic lupus erythematosus in NZB × NZW F1 mice treated with the testosterone-blocking drug flutamide. *J Lab Clin Med* 1994;**124**:401–7.

99 Angele MK, Wichmann MW, Ayala A, *et al*. Testosterone receptor blockade after hemorrhage in males. Restoration of the depressed immune functions and improved survival following subsequent sepsis. *Arch Surg* 1997;**132**:1207–14.

100 Furr BJ. The development of Casodex (bucalutamide): preclinical studies. *Eur Urol* 1996;**29**:83–95.

6: The adrenal in critical care – do we neglect this vital organ?

MURAD G GHREW, PAUL HOLLOWAY

Introduction

Virtually all patients admitted to an intensive care unit (ICU) can be assumed to be in a state of extreme stress. Although many routine diagnostic investigations are carried out, assessment of endocrine function is usually limited to clinical examination, supported by inferences from simple analyses such as electrolyte, acid–base and blood glucose measurement. In the absence of obvious clues to adrenal dysfunction, patients' management may proceed without further specific attention to this organ, despite the vital role of the adrenal in the response to stress. In the management of severe shock inotrope dependency may, in some circumstances, suggest inadequate capacity of the adrenal medulla to contribute to circulatory compensation, but this represents failure of only one of the adrenal's key functions.

The purpose of this article is to focus on the adrenal gland in critical care medicine, highlighting in particular the secondary effects of both critical illness and current intensive care therapies, on adrenal function. In addition, the means at our disposal for diagnosing adrenal dysfunction and to appropriate management will be discussed. We will not address in detail the management of primary overactivity of adrenal cortical function as this is not only rare, but seldom requires definable alterations in critical care management. As the adrenal does not function as an independent endocrine organ this will necessitate coverage of the relationship and dependency of the adrenal on the function of other organs, particularly the hypothalamus and pituitary. A recap of the range of homeostatic functions of the adrenal gland, and practical guidance on the evaluation and effective therapeutic compensation of adrenal function in critical care patients will also be provided.

What are the adrenal glands?

The adrenal glands are vital endocrine organs which can be divided on a histological basis into cortex and medulla, which specialise in producing different hormones. The adrenal medulla produces adrenaline (epinephrine) and noradrenaline (norepinephrine) in response to stress and sympathetic stimulation. Aldosterone is the major mineralocorticoid produced by the zona glomerulosa (outer zone). It promotes renal tubular reabsorption of sodium and excretion of potassium. Its secretion is regulated by the renin–angiotensin–aldosterone system but also influenced directly by hyperkalaemia, dopamine and atrial natriuretic peptide. Androgens produced by the zona fasciculata (inner zone) include dehydroepiandrosterone sulphate (DHEAS) and dehydroepiandrosterone (DHEA), testosterone and androstenedione.

Cortisol is the major glucocorticoid secreted by both the zona fasciculata and reticularis. Its secretion is controlled by the hypothalamic–pituitary–adrenal axis, which is also responsible for the normal diurnal variation. Cortisol has complex metabolic and anti-inflammatory actions (Box 6.1). It has a significant role in the maintenance of vascular tone, endothelial integrity, vascular permeability and the distribution of total body

---

Box 6.1 Physiological actions of glucocorticoids

- Increase hepatic glycogen and promote gluconeogenesis
- Suppress secretion of insulin
- Inhibit synthesis of nucleic acids in most tissues
- Inhibit protein synthesis and increase protein breakdown
- Enhance activation of cellular lipase by catecholamines
- Inhibit calcium uptake by renal tubules/gut, redistribute intracellular calcium
- Increase renal free-water clearance
- Maintain normal vascular responsiveness to vasoconstrictor agents
- Oppose inflammatory enhancement of capillary permeability
- Inhibit production and action of inflammatory mediators
- Inhibit production and function of interleukin-1 and interleukin-2
- Required for the production of angiotensin II
- Inhibit cytotoxic activity of natural killer (NK) cells
- Cause polymorphonuclear leucocytosis
- Redistribute eosinophils and lymphocytes

---

water. It also potentiates the vasoconstrictive action of catecholamines. All are vital for the ability of the body to cope with various degrees of stress. In normal subjects, the daily rate of cortisol production is estimated at 15.7 μmol per square metre of body surface area. During severe stress (e.g. major surgery) the adrenal gland in an adult can produce up to 828 μmol/24 h of cortisol. This is also accompanied by loss of diurnal variation. Serum cortisol levels correlate positively with the severity of the illness, thus the values are highest in patients with the highest illness severity scores. Values are very high shortly before death (828–7173 nmol/L).[1,2]

Adrenal cortex and critical illness

Acute adrenocortical insufficiency can present as a severe life-threatening illness also referred to as an adrenal or Addisonian crisis. More commonly, adrenal dysfunction or impairment of the hypothalamic–pituitary–adrenal axis only becomes an issue when patients already receiving corticosteroid therapy develop a severe illness or are subjected to severe stress such as major trauma or surgery. The pathophysiology of the systemic inflammatory response syndrome (SIRS) can include physiological rather than anatomical interference with adrenal function leading to transient hypoadrenalism.[3-5] A state in which corticosteroid therapy diminishes or eliminates the requirements for vasopressor drugs despite normal serum cortisol levels may occur in some critically ill patients and is often referred to as occult or relative adrenal insufficiency.[6,7]

Acute adrenal insufficiency

Acute adrenal insufficiency in a patient with previously unknown adrenal disorder is rare. Crises commonly occur in the course of chronically treated insufficiency and are more commonly seen in primary than secondary adrenal insufficiency. Box 6.2 lists some of the known causes, the commonest scenario being a patient on steroid replacement developing an acute illness or stress such that treatment is not taken.

The clinical manifestations of an adrenal crisis are variable and non-specific. Weakness, anorexia, nausea, vomiting, abdominal pain, fever, hyperpigmentation, vitiligo, hyponatraemia, hyperkalaemia, hypoglycaemia and eosinophilia in any combination should raise the suspicion of hypoadrenalism.[8,9] Spontaneous adrenal insufficiency due to adrenal haemorrhage and adrenal vein thrombosis must be considered in patients presenting with vomiting, abdominal pain, rigidity, confusion and hypotension. Laparotomy for a patient in adrenal crisis is likely to have a fatal outcome.

59

Box 6.2 Causes of adrenal crisis

- Sudden cessation of steroid therapy
- Severe stress (e.g. infection, trauma) in patients with chronic adrenal insufficiency
- Bilateral adrenal haemorrhage (e.g. meningococcal sepsis, pseudomonal sepsis, anticoagulant therapy)
- Adrenal vein thrombosis
- Acute secondary insufficiency (e.g. pituitary infarction, bleeding into pituitary tumour, postpartum pituitary necrosis)

Circulatory collapse in adrenal crises characteristically mimics hypovolaemic shock (decreased preload, depressed myocardial contractility and increased peripheral vascular resistance). It can also produce a clinical picture indistinguishable from septic shock with fever, hypotension, peripheral vasodilatation and high cardiac-output state. In primary adrenal insufficiency where mineralocorticoids are also deficient, the hypovolaemic picture is more likely. Patients who receive adequate fluid replacement are more likely to show hyperdynamic status.[1,10]

Classical biochemical abnormalities of adrenal hypofunction – hypoglycaemia, hyponatraemia, hyperkalaemia, metabolic acidosis (ketosis) and hypercalcaemia – which may all occur to variable degrees, should be considered as late complications of decompensation and thus indicators of the severity of disease. Whilst many of these should have been identified and evaluated prior to the patient's admission to the ICU, the stress during the admission episode may be the first opportunity for such abnormalities to become manifest. One example is relative hypoglycaemia (blood glucose within the fasting range) when the 'normal' range in a critically ill patient may extend into the diabetic range as a result of the normal glucocorticoid response to stress. Interpretation of electrolyte disturbances – low serum sodium with high potassium with converse urine levels – may be complicated by fluid and diuretic management but adrenal hypofunction should be excluded both in this situation and in all patients with persistent unexplained metabolic acidosis, particularly ketoacidosis, in the absence of hyperglycaemia.

Relative adrenal insufficiency

In recent years there have been several case reports where clinical and biochemical observations have indicated occult or relative adrenal insufficiency in critically ill patients.[6,7,11] Signs and symptoms that may give rise to suspicion include unexplained circulatory instability, discrepancy between the anticipated severity of the disease and the present state of the patient and high fever without apparent cause, and which does not respond to antibiotic therapy. There are no strict biochemical criteria for the diagnosis of relative adrenal insufficiency. Baseline serum cortisol levels and response to corticotrophin stimulation test may be within the normal limits but may be inappropriately low for the severity of the illness.

One possible explanation for this relative dysfunction is the pre-existence of subclinical hypoadrenalism, such that although the adrenal gland can produce enough steroids to cope with minor stresses, it is overwhelmed by more severe illness. Another possibility includes involvement of the adrenal glands in the disease process itself, either anatomically (e.g. haemorrhage) or functionally as part of the multiorgan failure syndrome. In addition, cytokine-mediated inhibition of corticotrophin release and the use of drugs that interfere with steroid synthesis, such as etomidate, may also offer an explanation.[3,12–14] Whether due to pre-existing subclinical adrenal disease, or as a feature of severe illness, relative adrenal insufficiency can be of clinical importance. Steroid replacement at maximum physiological doses (100–300 mg hydrocortisone per 24 hours) has been shown to reduce the vasopressor drug requirement and facilitate weaning from mechanical ventilation in the critically ill patient on ICU.[6]

Transient adrenal insufficiency

Transient hypoadrenalism as evidenced by subnormal basal and stimulated cortisol levels has been described in patients with SIRS.[5] Administration of physiological doses of hydrocortisone to these patients led to rapid decrease in temperature and improvement of haemodynamic status. Following recovery, all patients were successfully weaned off steroids and subsequent adrenal function tests were normal. This suggests that transient adrenal hypofunction can be a feature of SIRS, although the mechanism remains unclear and is likely to be multifactorial. SIRS is associated with the release of a range of inflammatory mediators. Most of these molecules stimulate steroidogenesis either indirectly by stimulating the hypothalamic–pituitary–adrenal axis – interleukin-1 (IL-1), IL-3, IL-6, IL-10 and tumour necrosis factor-α (TNF-α) – or directly, through stimulation of the adrenal cells (IL-2, IL-3, IL-6).[3,13–17] However, some mediators of the immune/inflammatory responses have also been shown to have suppressant effects on steroidogenesis, shown in Table 6.1. Interferon (IFN)-α2b reduces ACTH-induced production of cortisol by cultured adrenal cells.[18] Stimulated human lymphocytes produce fragments of ACTH molecules that may have some biological activity. Such peptides may interfere with ACTH binding to its receptor. Corticostatins have been shown to impair adrenal cortex function by competing with ACTH binding

Table 6.1 Factors influencing steroidogenesis at different levels of the hypothalamic–pituitary–adrenal system

Inhibitors of steroidogenesis	Stimulators of steroidogenesis
Hypothalamus	
Adrenocorticotrophin (ACTH)	Serotonin (5-HT)
γ-aminobutyric acid	Interleukins -1, -3, -6 and -10
β-endorphin	Tumour necrosis factor-α
Corticotrophin-releasing hormone	
Leptin	
Substance P	
Somatostatin	
Oxytocin	
Nitric oxide	
Carbon monoxide	
Lipocortin-1	
Glucocorticoids	
Endorphins	
Pituitary	
Atrial natriuretic peptide	Corticotrophin-releasing hormone
Thyroid-releasing hormone	Arginine-vasopressin
Lipocortin-1	
Adrenomedulin	
Adrenal	
Corticostatins	Adrenocorticotrophin (ACTH)
Transforming growth factor-β	Interleukins -2, -3 and -6
Interferon-α2b	Catecholamines
ACTH-related peptides	Neuropeptide Y
	Migration inhibitory factor
	Endothelins

to its receptor. The plasma level of these peptides, produced by neutrophils and cells of myeloid lineage, increases during infection in animals.[3,19]

In fact, the distinction between transient and relative adrenal insufficiency is dependent only on the cut-off point above which basal and stimulated cortisol levels are considered to be normal. 'Reference interval' blood cortisol levels in critical illness are not well documented and various studies have adopted levels between >100 nmol/L and >500 nmol/L as cut-off points.[4] Naturally the higher the cut-off point used the more likely it is that adrenal hypofunction is diagnosed. The reported incidence of hypoadrenalism in septic shock varies between 3 and 52% depending on the definition used. As in general medicine there is limited value in 'random' serum cortisol measurement but in critical care an expected surge in ACTH release, together with contributions from the SIRS response as mentioned, should stimulate the adrenal cortex sufficiently to allow blood cortisol levels to rise towards the top end of this range (i.e. one would expect values >500 nmol/L) in most patients at admission. Because of the variability of 'random cortisol' a dynamic adrenocortical stimulation test is indicated and in most instances the short Synacthen test is adequate. There is current discussion in the literature about the relative merits of the high dose, supraphysiological (250 μ) and low-dose (1 μ) Synacthen test in assessing the hypothalamic–pituitary–adrenal axis, but the most compelling evidence suggests that the latter has better predictive value and also has benefits over the insulin hypoglycaemia test as an alternative.[20,21] Either Synacthen test can be performed with ease and without risk in critical care patients and should be carried out whenever adrenal hypofunction is suspected. A rise in serum cortisol above 580 nmol/L by 30 minutes excludes the diagnosis of primary adrenal insufficiency. Non-ICU patients can have their adrenal stress response capacity evaluated by a longer stimulation test such as that provided by an 8 hour infusion of ACTH but this would seldom be viable or practical in ICU.

Corticosteroid therapy and replacement

Although corticosteroids are well-established adjunctive treatment for some critical conditions, e.g. *Pneumocystis carinii* pneumonia, the role of corticosteroids in critically ill patients with normal hypothalamic–pituitary–adrenal axes remains controversial. The results of clinical studies evaluating the use of steroids in sepsis and SIRS have been disappointing. However, corticosteroids might be beneficial in some circumstances. There is some evidence suggesting that steroids may be beneficial in the chronic fibroproliferative stage of acute respiratory distress syndrome.[22–24] Some evidence exists for the benefit of corticosteroids in bacterial meningitis especially severe tuberculous meningitis and *H. influenzae* meningitis in children.[25]

When the hypothalamic–pituitary–adrenal axis is abnormal, steroid-replacement therapy is vital. If hypoadrenalism is strongly suspected in a critically ill patient, corticosteroids should be started without delay after a blood sample is taken for baseline cortisol measurement. A short Synacthen test can be done at the same time but the initial steroid administered must be dexamethasone as this will not interfere with the test performance. More commonly, patients are already on steroid replacement or therapy when they are admitted with critical illness. Patients known to have hypoadrenalism on steroid replacement should ideally be changed to a continuous hydrocortisone infusion at maximum physiological dosage (100–300 mg). Similar doses can be given as a replacement for patients with impaired hypothalamic–pituitary–adrenal axis as a result of prolonged steroid therapy, e.g. for autoimmune disease. Special situations may arise if corticosteroid treatment has been discontinued recently. High dose and prolonged treatment do not invariably correlate with the degree and duration of hypothalamic–pituitary–adrenal suppression.[1] It is important for the intensivist to remember that after long-term glucocorticoid therapy, recovery of the suppressed adrenal response may take more than one year, and the low-dose corticotrophin test can detect suppressed adrenal response even in patients who have recently received glucocorticoid therapy for periods as short as 5 days.[26]

Adrenal medulla and critical illness

Underactivity

Primary or secondary underactivity of the adrenal medulla is seldom, if ever, an identifiable clinical entity and there is little literature describing such a phenomenon. Medullary dysfunction is implied in the context of primary hypoadrenalism but measurement of serum or urinary catecholamines or their metabolites to look for underactivity would be unhelpful in clinical practice, particularly in critical care, where the contribution from extra-adrenal paraneuronal and paraganglial tissues may be significant. Failure of the adrenal medullary response to stress may be implied in some cases of unexplained shock when large doses of catecholamines or their analogues are required to sustain viable circulatory function.

Overactivity: Phaeochromocytoma

Phaeochromocytomas are rare chromaffin cell tumours arising predominantly in the adrenal medulla but may also develop from chromaffin cells elsewhere in the sympathetic ganglia. Predisposition to development of a tumour can be inherited as an autosomal dominant trait, either alone or in combination with other abnormalities such as multiple endocrine neoplasia (MEN) type IIa and IIb, neurofibromatosis and Von Hippel–Lindau syndrome. Tumour cells produce, store and secrete a variety of peptides including adrenaline, noradrenaline, dopamine, endogenous opioids, neuropeptide Y, chromagranin A, parathyroid hormone (PTH)-like peptide and erythropoietin. Increased release of most of these peptides have little clinical significance and it is the excessive catecholamine production which is the cause of the symptoms and complications of phaeochromocytoma. Most patients with phaeochromocytoma come to medical attention as a result of hypertensive crises or during investigation of labile hypertension resistant to treatment. Some do, however, present with sustained hypertension or acute left ventricular failure. Patients may present with paroxysmal symptoms of headache, anxiety, apprehension, profuse sweating, chest or abdominal pain, pallor or flushing during the paroxysm. Despite improved diagnostic techniques over recent years, at least 50% of these tumours are diagnosed for the first time at postmortem.

Intensivists may encounter phaeochromocytoma in several clinical scenarios and patients can present with severe haemodynamic instability ranging from hypertensive crisis to a state of shock due to tumour haemorrhage or infarction. Severe hypotension or shock can be precipitated by major trauma or surgery in patients with undiagnosed phaeochromocytoma, due to severe volume collapse and blunted sympathetic reflexes. For the same reasons, patients undergoing surgery for phaeochromocytoma need careful pre-operative preparation with adequate α- and β-blockade and volume replacement and also may need a period of postoperative intensive care. Unusual, but known presentations, include an acute abdomen due to a ruptured tumour, hyperamylasaemia and multiorgan failure mimicking pancreatitis, myocardial infarction with normal coronaries and myocarditis/cardiomyopathy.[27-29] Paroxysms of crisis can be precipitated with a variety of drugs such as opiates, metoclopramide, tricyclic antidepressants and glucagon. A paroxysm of hypertension and anxiety following administration of any of these drugs should raise the suspicion of occult disease.

Hypertensive crisis can initially be controlled with continuous intravenous nitroprusside or phentolamine. Vasodilator therapy will reveal the presence of volume depletion and the patient will often need resuscitation with large volumes of fluid. Intravenous infusion of a beta-blocker (e.g. esmolol) can be used to control tachyarrhythmias but should not be infused alone, to avoid precipitation of hypertensive crises due to unopposed beta-stimulation. Severe circulatory collapse due to tumour infarction needs aggressive volume replacement and inotropic/vasopressor support, sometimes in very high doses, to combat receptor downregulation.

Blood analysis may reveal a high haematocrit due to haemoconcentration and volume depletion, but rarely can be due to production of erythropoietin. Catecholamines are diabetogenic hormones that suppress insulin secretion and accelerate hepatic gluconeogenesis. Impaired glucose tolerance is a feature of phaeochromocytoma in up to 50% of patients. Hypercalcaemia can be induced by a PTH-like peptide produced by the tumour but its presence should raise the suspicion of multiple endocrine neoplasia syndrome. Hypokalaemia may also occur from transient potassium influx into cells.

Assay of urinary catecholamines or their metabolites, metanephrines and vanillylmandelic acid (VMA), in an acidified 24-hour collection of urine taken during or immediately following episodic attack can detect most phaeochromocytomas.[30] Interpretation of raised urine catecholamine levels

65

in critical care patients need to be discussed with chemical pathologists who would normally insist on three separate collections in equivocal cases. Plasma adrenaline, noradrenaline or dopamine levels are always raised during and immediately following paroxysms but basal levels can be normal.[31] Again interpretation of random serum catecholamine levels in ICU patients is complex and should only be contemplated in anuric patients. The time scale for analysis will often delay diagnosis and prior discussion with the laboratory is essential. Computed tomography scan and MRI are very helpful in confirmation and localisation of the tumour. MIBG scans can help localise the tumour with high sensitivity (85%) and specificity (90%).

Surgical removal of the tumour is feasible laparoscopically in most patients and if done before cardiovascular damage occurs, complete cure can be expected. Surgery should be preceded by optimal α-blockade with phenoxybenzamine (supine BP <160/90 mmHg and standing BP >80/45 mmHg). β-Blockade can be added following α-blockade to control reflex tachycardia or dysrrhythmia. Intraoperative volume replacement should be given generously.

Conclusions

Adrenal dysfunction is relatively common in critical care patients and there is a strong argument for routine assessment of the hypothalamic–pituitary–adrenal axis in all patients admitted for intensive care. This review has highlighted some of the mechanisms for adrenal dysfunction in critical care and the diagnostic techniques available for clinical use. Further clinical trials of adrenal supportive therapy are needed to guide appropriate management.

References

1 SW Lamberts, Bruining HA, De Jong FH. Corticosteroid therapy in severe illness. *N Engl J Med* 1997;**337**:1285–91.
2 Wade CE, Lindberg JS, Cockrell JL, *et al.* Upon-admission adrenal steroidogenesis is adapted to the degree of illness in intensive care unit patients. *J Clin Endocrinol Metab* 1988;**67**:223–7.
3 Soni A, Pepper GM, Wyrwinski PM, *et al.* Adrenal insufficiency occurring during septic shock: incidence, outcome, and relationship to peripheral cytokine levels. *Am J Med* 1995;**98**:266–71.
4 Hatherill M, Tibby SM, Hilliard T, *et al.* Adrenal insufficiency in septic shock. *Arch Dis Child* 1999;**80**:51–5.
5 Mackenzie JS, Burrows L, Burchard KW. Transient hypoadrenalism during surgical critical illness. *Arch Surg* 1998;**133**:199–204.

6   Baldwin WA, Allo M. Occult hypoadrenalism in critically ill patients. *Arch Surg* 1993;**128**:673–6.

7   Ligtenberg JJ, Van der Werf TS, Tulleken JE, *et al.* Diagnosis of relative adrenal insufficiency in critically ill patients. *Lancet* 1999;**354**:774–5.

8   Angelis M, Yu M, Takanishi D, *et al.* Eosinophilia as a marker of adrenal insufficiency in the surgical intensive care unit. *J Am Coll Surg* 1996;**183**:589–96.

9   Oelkers W. Adrenal insufficiency. *N Engl J Med* 1996;**335**:1206–11.

10 Dorin RI, Kearns PJ. High cardiac output circulatory failure in acute adrenal insufficiency. *Crit Care Med* 1988;**16**:296–7.

11 Caplan RH, Wickus G, Reynertson RH, Kisken WA. Occult hypoadrenalism in critically ill patients. *Arch Surg* 1994;**129**:456.

12 Wagner RL, White PF, Kan PB, *et al.* Inhibition of adrenal steroidogenesis by the anaesthetic etomidate. *N Engl J Med* 1984;**310**:1415–21.

13 Marx C, Ehrhart-Bornstein M, Scherbaum WA, Bornstein SR. Regulation of adrenocortical function by cytokines – relevance for immune–endocrine interaction. *Horm Metab Res* 1998;**30**:416–20.

14 Bornstein SR, Chrousos GP. Adrenocorticotropin (ACTH) and non-ACTH mediated regulation of the adrenal cortex: neural and immune inputs. *J Clin Endocrinol Metab* 1999;**84**:1729–36.

15 Judd AM. Cytokine expression in the rat adrenal cortex. *Horm Metab Res* 1998;**30**:404–10.

16 Path G, Bornstein SR, Ehrhart-Bornstein M, Scherbaum WA. Interleukin-6 and the interleukin-6 receptor in the human adrenal gland: expression and effects on steroidogenesis. *J Clin Endocrinol Metab* 1997;**82**:2343–9.

17 Path G, Bornstein SR, Spath-Schwalbe E, Scherbaum WA. Direct effects of interleukin-6 on human adrenal cells. *Endocr Res* 1996;**22**:867–73.

18 Tachikawa E, Itho K, Kudo K, *et al.* Effects of interferons on cortisol production in bovine adrenal fasciculata cells stimulated by adrenocorticotropin. *J Pharm Pharmacol* 1999;**51**:465–73.

19 Tominaga T, Fukata J, Hayashi Y, *et al.* Distribution and characterisation of immunoreactive corticostatin in the hypothalamic–pituitary–adrenal axis. *Endocrinology* 1992;**130**:1593–8.

20 Rasmuson S, Olsson T, Hagg E. A low dose ACTH test to assess the function of the hypothalamic–pituitary–adrenal axis. *Clin Endocrinol* 1996;**44**:151–6.

21 Hurel SJ, Thompson CJ, Watson MJ, *et al.* The short Synacthen and insulin stress tests in the assessment of the hypothalamic–pituitary–adrenal axis. *Clin Endocrinol* 1996;**44**:141–6.

22 Keel JB, Hauser M, Stocker R, *et al.* Established acute respiratory distress syndrome: benefit of corticosteroid rescue therapy. *Respiration* 1998;**65**:258–64.

23 Hooper RG, Kearl RA, Charles E. Established adult respiratory distress syndrome successfully treated with corticosteroids. *South Med J* 1996;**89**:359–64.

24 Biffl WL, Moore FA, Moore EE, *et al.* Are corticosteroids salvage therapy for refractory acute respiratory distress syndrome? *Am J Surg* 1995;**170**:591–5.

25 Coyle PK. Glucocorticoids in central nervous system bacterial infection. *Arch Neurol* 1999;**56**:796–801.

26 Henzen C, Suter A, Lerch E, *et al.* Suppression and recovery of adrenal response after short-term high dose glucocorticoid treatment. *Lancet* 2000;**355**:542–5.

27 Ong KL, Tan TH. Ruptured phaeochromocytoma – a rare differential diagnosis of acute abdomen. *Singapore Med J* 1996;**37**:113–14.
28 Ferguson Kl. Imipramine provoked paradoxical pheochromocytoma crisis. *Am J Emerg Med* 1994;**12**:190–2.
29 Gan TJ, Miller RF, Webb AR, Russell RC. Phaeochromocytoma presenting as acute hyperamylasaemia and multiorgan failure. *Can J Anaesth* 1994;**41**:244–7.
30 Tierney LM, McPhee SJ, Papadakis MA. Phaeochromocytoma. *CMDT 1999*, 38th edn, 1102–4.
31 Mannelli M, Ianni L, Cilotti A, Conti A. *et al*. Phaeochromocytoma in Italy: a multicentre retrospective study. *Eur J Endocrinol* 1999;**141**:619–24.